IMAGING ATLAS

OF THE NORMAL GALLBLADDER AND ITS VARIANTS

Edited by
Jon W. Meilstrup, M.D.
Assistant Professor
Chief, Diagnostic Ultrasound
The Pennsylvania State University
The Milton S. Hershey Medical Center
Hershey, Pennsylvania

CRC Press
Boca Raton Ann Arbor London Tokyo

Library of Congress Cataloging-in-Publication Data

Imaging atlas of the normal gallbladder and its variants / edited by Jon W. Meilstrup.
p. cm.
Includes bibliographical references and index.
ISBN 0–8493–4788–2
1. Gallbladder—Imaging—Atlases.
[DNLM: 1. Gallbladder—anatomy & histology—atlases.
2. Diagnostic Imaging—atlases. WI 17 I31 1994]
QM352.I46 1994
616.365′07572—dc20
DNLM/DLC
for Library of Congress 93–44006
CIP

Direct all inquiries to CRC Press, Inc., 2000 Corporate Blvd., N.W., Boca Raton, Florida 33431.

International Standard Book Number 0–8493–4788–2
Library of Congress Card Number 93–44006
Printed in the United States of America 1 2 3 4 5 6 7 8 9 0
Printed on acid-free paper

ACKNOWLEDGMENTS

I am grateful to all who have assisted in this endeavor—Marsha Baker and Monique Power of CRC Press, John E. Madewell, M.D., who has consistently given encouragement and support as chairman of radiology, and all of the sonographers, technologists, and residents who over the years have found and shared interesting gallbladder cases.

I am especially indebted to each of the several contributors who have made this monograph possible. Their expertise and interest have been invaluable. I would particularly like to thank two of my colleagues, Claudia Kasales, M.D., and Kenneth D. Hopper, M.D., who collaborated with me on several chapters, and who have given so much in the way of time, encouragement, suggestions, and help.

I am grateful for the secretarial support of Doreen Katzaman, and especially for my secretary, Mary Bihl, who attended so well to the many details and revisions.

And, finally, I appreciate the constant support and encouragement of my wife and family.

Jon W. Meilstrup, M.D.
Hershey, Pennsylvania

THE EDITOR

Jon W. Meilstrup, M.D., is Chief of Diagnostic Ultrasound, Department of Radiology, The Pennsylvania State University, The Milton S. Hershey Medical Center, Hershey, Pennsylvania.

Dr. Meilstrup graduated in 1970 from the University of Utah, Salt Lake City, Utah, with a Bachelor of Music degree in organ performance (*magna cum laude*) and obtained his M.D. degree in 1976 from the University of Utah School of Medicine. He completed his residency training at the University of Missouri-Columbia Medical Center in 1980. He was Officer in Charge of Ultrasound at Walter Reed Army Medical Center from 1981 to 1985, and Officer in Charge of Imaging (CT-US) from 1983 to 1985.

Dr. Meilstrup is a member of the American College of Radiology, Radiological Society of North America, American Roentgen Ray Society, American Institute of Ultrasound in Medicine, Association of University Radiologists, Pennsylvania Radiological Society, Society of Radiologists in Ultrasound, and Society of Vascular Technology.

Dr. Meilstrup has current research interests in various aspects of upper abdominal imaging, including the evaluation of periportal lucency on computed tomography as a possible normal variant. He has eight published articles, has had material presented at four national meetings, and has given many local and regional lectures and presentations. He has helped to produce exhibits shown in 19 national or state medical meetings, 3 of these winning second place awards.

Dr. Meilstrup is married and has eight children, and lives in the Hershey, Pennsylvania area.

CONTRIBUTORS

Abraham Dachman, M.D.
Associate Professor
Chief, Abdominal Imaging
Director, Computed Tomography
The University of Chicago
Chicago, Illinois

Kenneth D. Hopper, M.D.
Associate Professor of Radiology
Chief, Body Imaging/Radiology Research
The Pennsylvania State University
Hershey, Pennsylvania

Claudia J. Kasales, M.D.
Assistant Professor of Radiology
The Pennsylvania State University
Hershey, Pennsylvania

Rickhesvar Mahraj, F.R.C.R.
Assistant Professor of Radiology
Academic Director of Chest Radiology
The Pennsylvania State University
Hershey, Pennsylvania

Carson Schneck, M.D.
Professor of Anatomy and Diagnostic Imaging
Temple University School of Medicine
Philadelphia, Pennsylvania

Gary A. Thieme, M.D.
Associate Professor of Radiology
University of Colorado School of Medicine
Denver, Colorado

Simon Westacott, F.R.C.R.
Assistant Professor of Radiology
The Pennsylvania State University
Hershey, Pennsylvania

TABLE OF CONTENTS

IMAGING ATLAS

OF THE NORMAL GALLBLADDER AND ITS VARIANTS

Chapter 1

INTRODUCTION

Jon W. Meilstrup

It is not surprising that the gallbladder, a small sac-like structure which serves as the biliary reservoir, has been the source of so much discussion in recent years. Fifteen million Americans have gallstones,[1] many of which are asymptomatic.[2] With this potential cause of significant morbidity, it is no wonder there is interest in the gallbladder and the diagnosis of gallbladder disease.

Since 1900, when gallstones were first radiographically detected, continual improvement has taken place in gallbladder imaging.[3] The development of contrast media led to oral cholecystography, and with additional technological advances, sonography became available. While they have limited roles in specifically imaging the gallbladder, computed tomography (CT) and magnetic resonance imaging (MRI) are frequently used to evaluate the abdomen, including the gallbladder. Recently, percutaneous intraluminal gallbladder ultrasound has even been reported as a diagnostic tool.[4] New therapies for gallbladder disease, such as chemical dissolution of gallstones, lithotripsy, laparoscopic cholecystectomy, and percutaneous cholecystostomy and drainage attest to the continued need for appropriate imaging and diagnosis in gallbladder disease. Vital to current clinical workup and correct diagnosis is a knowledge of the wide array of normal gallbladder appearances, variants, mimics, and artifacts.

This volume deals with the range of appearances of the normal gallbladder and its variants. A discussion of anatomy, embryology, and imaging techniques is included for a better understanding of the normal gallbladder. Variants are grouped into three categories: anomalies of number, location, and form,[5] each addressed in a separate chapter. Discussions of imaging artifacts of the gallbladder and pseudolesions which can mimic gallbladder disease are also included. A short chapter on the appearance of the fetal gallbladder is provided for completeness. Biliary duct variants are not treated here, except where they relate to a specific gallbladder entity.

Because sonography and CT are so frequently used to evaluate the gallbladder and upper abdomen, variants seen with these modalities are emphasized throughout this volume. However, other imaging modalities such as oral cholecystography, endoscopic retrograde cholecystopancreatography (ERCP), scintigraphy, and MRI are also included.

The case examples used in this volume have been largely collected by the editor and contributors because of their particular fascination with the

0-8493-4788-2/94/$0.00+$.50

variable appearance of the normal gallbladder. As various imaging modalities have developed, we have been excited to see the gallbladder displayed to new and different advantages. When viewing gallbladder imaging studies, especially when an unusual variant is evident, each image must be carefully evaluated against a backdrop of knowledge of what is normal and what is not. We believe that ". . . improvement in the accuracy of differential diagnosis resulting from the more effective use of normal findings should improve patient care by aiding in the process of making sound decisions."[6]

To this end, it is hoped that the reader finds a similar interest in the many gallbladder variants that inevitably will be seen in clinical practice, and that this small volume will help the reader in making an appropriate clinical diagnosis when imaging the normal gallbladder.

REFERENCES

1. **Kalser, M. H.,** Cholelithiasis: clinical aspects, in *Bockus Gastroenterology*, 4th ed., Berk, J. E., Haubrich, W. S., Kalser, M. H., Roth, J. L. A., and Schaffner, F., Eds., W. B. Saunders, Philadelphia, 1985, 3619.
2. **Hopper, K. D., Landis, J. R., Meilstrup, J. W., McCauslin, M. A., and Sechtin, A. G.,** The prevalence of asymptomatic gallstones in the general population, *Invest. Radiol.*, 26, 939, 1991.
3. **Feld, R., Kurtz, A. B., and Zeman, R. K.,** Imaging the gallbladder: a historical perspective, *AJR*, 156, 737, 1991.
4. **van Sonnenberg, E., D'Agostino, H. B., Sanchez, R. L., Goodacre, B. B., Esch, O. G., Easter, D. E., and Gosink, B. B.,** Percutaneous intraluminal US in the gallbladder and bile ducts, *Radiology*, 182, 693, 1992.
5. **Lockwood, B. C.,** Congenital anomalies of the gallbladder, *JAMA*, 136, 678, 1948.
6. **Gorry, G. A., Pauker, S. G., and Schwartz, W. B.,** The diagnostic importance of the normal finding, *N. Engl. J. Med.*, 298, 486, 1978.

Chapter 2

NORMAL GALLBLADDER ANATOMY AND IMAGING

Simon Westacott and Rickhesvar Mahraj

TABLE OF CONTENTS

0–8493–4788–2/94/$0.00+$.50

I. INTRODUCTION

This chapter defines the most common arrangement of the gross anatomy of the gallbladder, including its relations and vascular anatomy, gives a short account of its microscopic structure, and describes the appearance of these structures when imaged by different modalities.

II. NORMAL ANATOMY

The gallbladder is a pear-shaped, hollow viscus (Figure 1) that is connected to the extrahepatic biliary tree by the cystic duct. Bile from the hepatocytes is stored and concentrated in the gallbladder and ultimately ejected into the gastrointestinal (GI) tract, under the influence of the parasympathetic nervous system and circulating hormones, notably cholecystokinin. There is considerable variation in dimensions; approximate length and diameter of the fully distended gallbladder are 10 and 4 cm, respectively. The gallbladder's capacity is up to 45 ml.[1]

The gallbladder is divided into a fundus, body, and neck. The fundus is a hemispherical ending which forms the anteroinferior margin. The neck forms the posterosuperior limit of the gallbladder and connects it to the cystic duct. The gallbladder lumen is widest at the junction of the body and the fundus and tapers toward the neck; the most rapidly tapering segment is called the infundibulum. Hartmann's pouch is a pathological saccular expansion of the neck and not a feature of normal anatomy.[2]

The gallbladder is located in the gallbladder fossa,[3] a concavity of the inferior surface of the liver which generally marks the caudal limit of the interlobar fissure* separating the right and left hepatic lobes. The body and neck are loosely attached to the liver by connective tissue, which is continuous with the connective tissue of the interlobar fissure. Peritoneum covers the fundus, which frequently projects beyond the inferior margin of the liver, and those parts of the gallbladder not directly adherent to the liver. The degree of contact between the gallbladder and the liver is highly variable: in some individuals the gallbladder is invaginated into the interlobar fissure; conversely, it may be entirely enveloped by peritoneum, in which case it is attached to the liver by a mesentery.

The gallbladder fossa is continuous posterosuperiorly with the porta hepatis, a transverse groove in the inferior surface of the liver traversed by the hepatic artery, portal vein, and common bile duct. A reflection of the peritoneum which covers the inferior surface of the liver forms a sleeve around these structures known as the hepatoduodenal ligament (free edge of the lesser omentum). Occasionally, a fold of peritoneum may connect the hepatoduodenal ligament to the peritoneal reflections around the gallbladder, forming the cholecystoduodenal ligament.

*The "true" or embryological interlobar fissure, within which the middle hepatic vein runs.

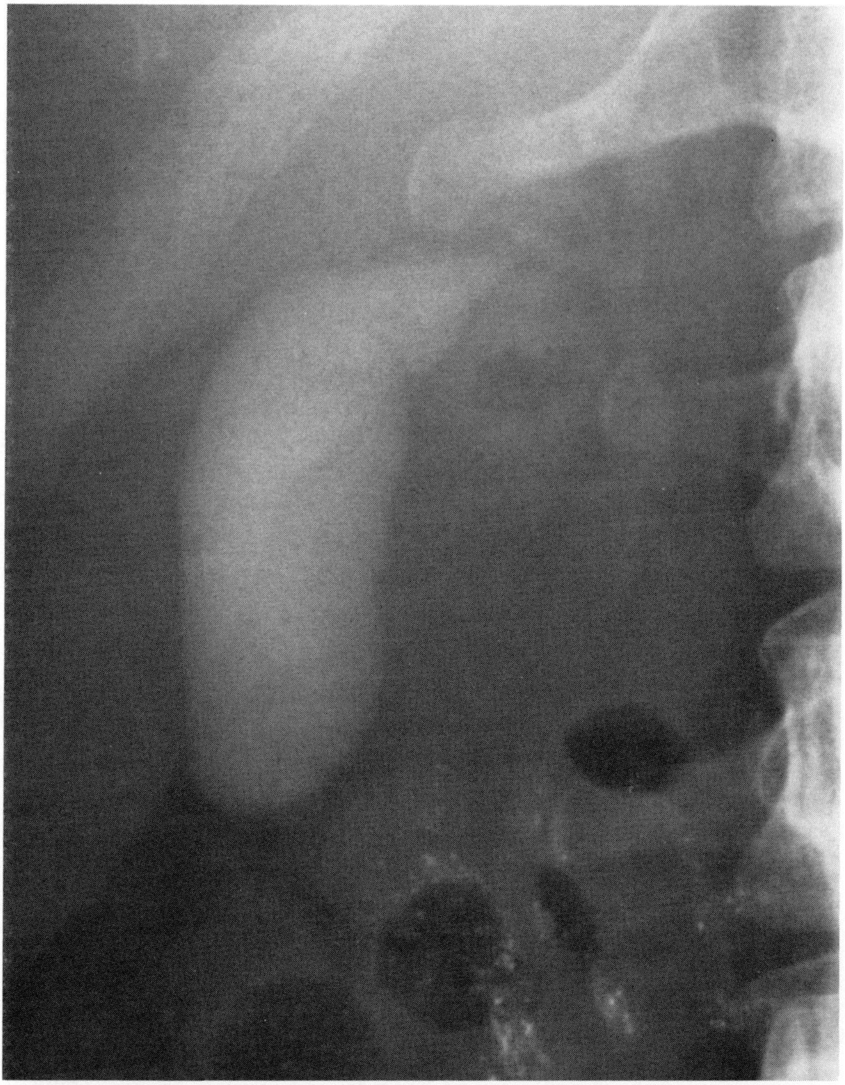

FIGURE 1. Oral cholecystogram demonstrating normal opacification of the gallbladder. Unabsorbed contrast remains in the transverse colon.

A. Connections and Relations

The gallbladder is connected to the biliary tree by the cystic duct, which joins the common hepatic duct to form the common bile duct. Anteriorly, the fundus of the gallbladder is related to the parietal peritoneum of the anterior abdominal wall; its surface marking is the junction of the costal margin with the lateral border of the rectus abdominis muscle. Antero-superiorly, the body of the gallbladder is in close contact with the liver.

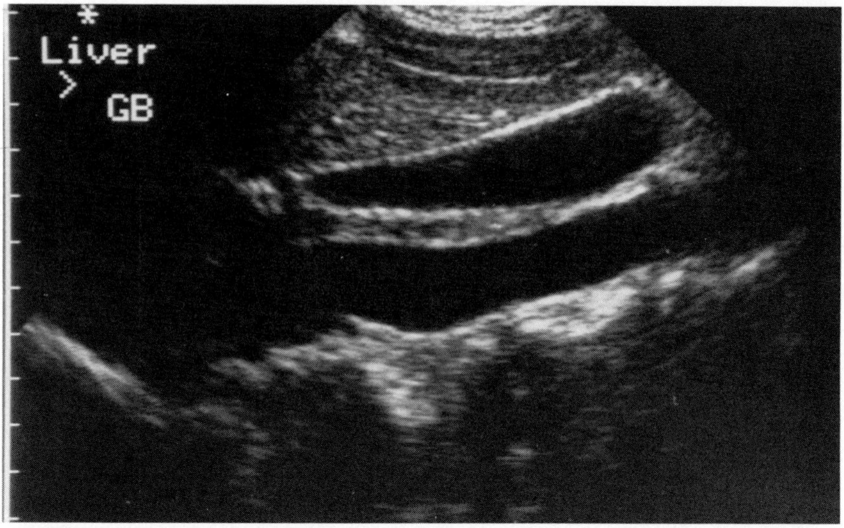

FIGURE 2. Longitudinal sonogram through a normal gallbladder.

Posteroinferiorly, the gallbladder is related to the second part of the duodenum and the transverse colon and, occasionally, to the inferior vena cava (Figure 2).

B. Vascular Supply

The arterial supply of the gallbladder emanates from the cystic artery, most commonly a branch of the right hepatic artery. Venous drainage is by multiple, small, unnamed vessels into the portal venous system. Lymphatic drainage is to nodes in the porta hepatis and subsequently to preaortic nodes near the celiac axis.

C. Histology

The gallbladder wall has three distinct layers. The outermost (serosal) layer is the peritoneum, as described above. The serosa is deficient in the areas in which the gallbladder is in contact with the liver, where it is replaced by connective tissue. Microscopic biliary radicles (ducts of Luschka), which arise from intrahepatic bile ducts, may extend into this connective tissue.[4] The innermost (mucosal) layer comprises columnar epithelium, which has both absorptive and mucus-secreting functions. The mucosa is raised into fine folds, more pronounced when the gallbladder is contracted. Outpouchings of mucosa through the outer layers produce Rokitansky-Aschoff sinuses which, although associated with disease, may be found in a significant proportion of normal adults.[4] The mucosa of the gallbladder is continuous with the mucosa of the cystic duct, where it is raised into spiral folds (valves of Heister). The intervening layer, the muscularis, comprises bundles of smooth muscle fibers oriented in circular, longitudinal, and oblique directions and encased in connective tissue. The muscularis continues into the wall of the cystic duct but not of the bile ducts.

III. IMAGING THE NORMAL GALLBLADDER

The normal anatomy of the gallbladder may be demonstrated using the imaging techniques that have been developed to examine diseases of the gallbladder. These include oral cholecystography, sonography, scintigraphy, computed tomography (CT), and magnetic resonance imaging (MRI). These complementary modalities reveal different aspects of the gallbladder to advantage.

A. Oral Cholecystography

Oral cholecystography utilizes contrast agents which are triiodinated benzene ring derivatives.[5] These agents require proper gastrointestinal absorption and adequate liver function to conjugate the contrast agent with glucuronide in the liver prior to excretion into bile. The concentration of the contrast agent in the gallbladder requires a patent cystic duct and functioning gallbladder mucosa. Such accumulation of contrast in the gallbladder gives a good demonstration of the lumen of the normal gallbladder and cystic duct (Figure 1). Because of the greater density of the contrast agent compared to bile, imaging with the patient in different positions will display different portions of the gallbladder. The fundus, therefore, is best seen in the erect and prone positions, the body in the prone and supine positions, and the neck in the supine position.

The size and shape of the fasting gallbladder can be assessed, including the presence of folds and septations. Contraction of the gallbladder following a fatty meal may give improved views of the cystic duct and may better demonstrate Rokitansky-Aschoff sinuses.

B. Sonography

Imaging is commonly performed using electronically focused, phased-array transducers between 3 and 5 MHz. The normal gallbladder should be visualized in nearly all patients after an 8 to 12 hour fast. Both the size and location are easily assessed in all planes. The relationship of the gallbladder to surrounding structures and the fixed relationship of the neck of the gallbladder to the main lobar fissure and the undivided right portal vein can be easily seen.[3] Unlike oral cholecystography, sonography is able to demonstrate the gallbladder wall. This is seen as a thin, echogenic stripe, 1 to 3 mm thick. Differentiation of the separate layers of the wall of the distended gallbladder is not possible, though folds, septations, and redundant mucosa in the contracted gallbladder can be seen.[6] The valves of Heister occasionally can be seen as linear echoes in the region of the cystic duct. Normal bile is echo-free and gives the gallbladder its characteristic cystic appearance on sonography (Figure 2).

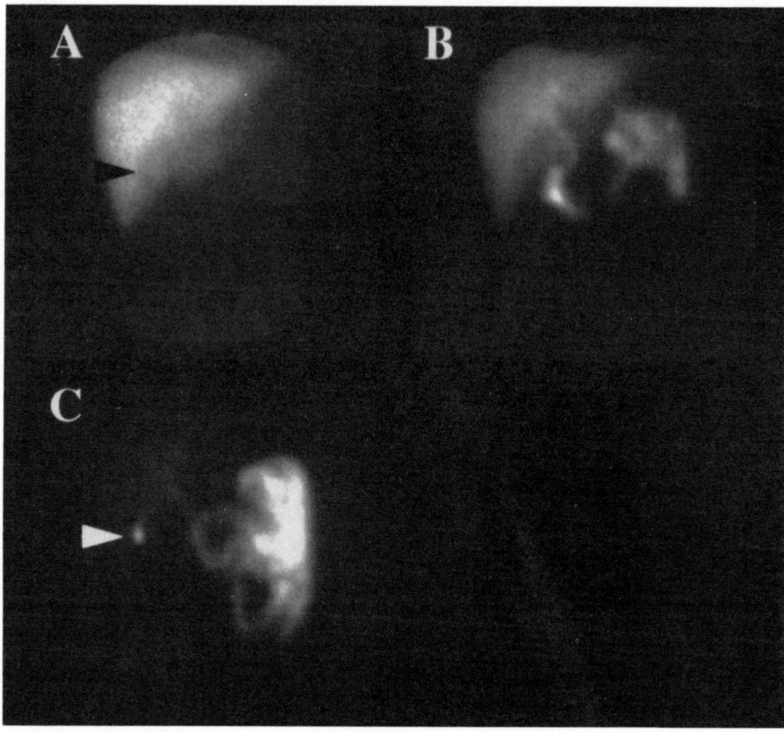

FIGURE 3. ^{99m}Tc mebrofenin biliary radionuclide scan. The immediate image (A) demonstrates hepatic parenchymal uptake and residual blood pool activity. A photo deficient area (black arrowhead) corresponds to the gallbladder fossa. An image taken 10 minutes after injection (B) demonstrates uptake in the biliary tree and small bowel. An image taken 30 minutes after injection (C) demonstrates activity in the gallbladder (white arrowhead) and small bowel, with ''wash-out'' from the liver. (Courtesy of Mark Tulchinsky, M.D.)

C. Scintigraphy

Nuclear imaging is commonly performed using technetium-labeled iminodiacetic acid analogues. When 5 mCi of this radiopharmaceutical are injected intravenously, the agent is excreted into bile without conjugation and accumulates in the normal gallbladder within 30 minutes. This form of imaging is designed to assess patency of the cystic duct and gives poor anatomic information. It demonstrates the lumen of the gallbladder, showing its location in relation to the liver and biliary tree (Figure 3). In

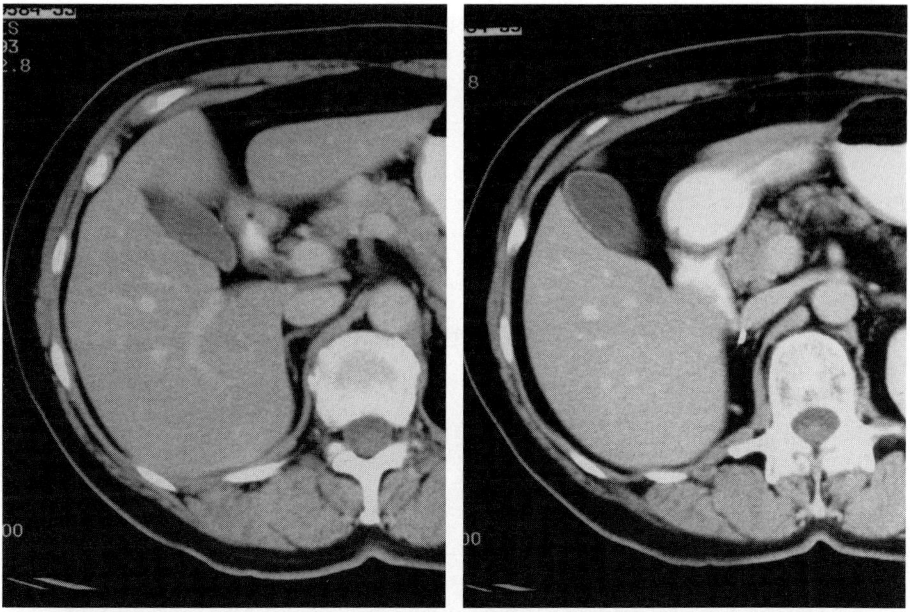

FIGURE 4. Axial, enhanced CT images through the gallbladder neck (A) and fundus (B).

the normal population, despite a patent cystic duct, a small percentage of normal gallbladders fails to fill. With the use of delayed scans and intravenous morphine this limitation can be overcome. No significant information is obtained regarding folds or septations within the gallbladder; none is obtained regarding wall structure.

D. Computed Tomography

Computed tomography differentiates the wall and contents of the normal gallbladder. Following contrast enhancement, both the cystic artery and the gallbladder wall may be better demonstrated. Clear visualization of the neck of the gallbladder and junctional fold (a fold between the infundibulum and the neck of the gallbladder, commonly demonstrated by sonography) is not usually possible because of the ability of CT to scan only in the axial plane. However, the relationship of the gallbladder to the liver, interlobar fissure, and bowel is well depicted (Figure 4).

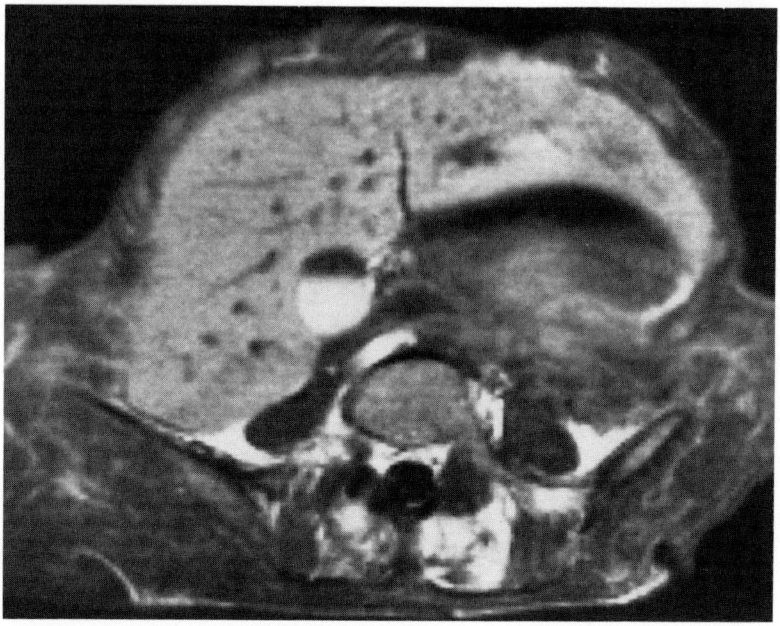

A

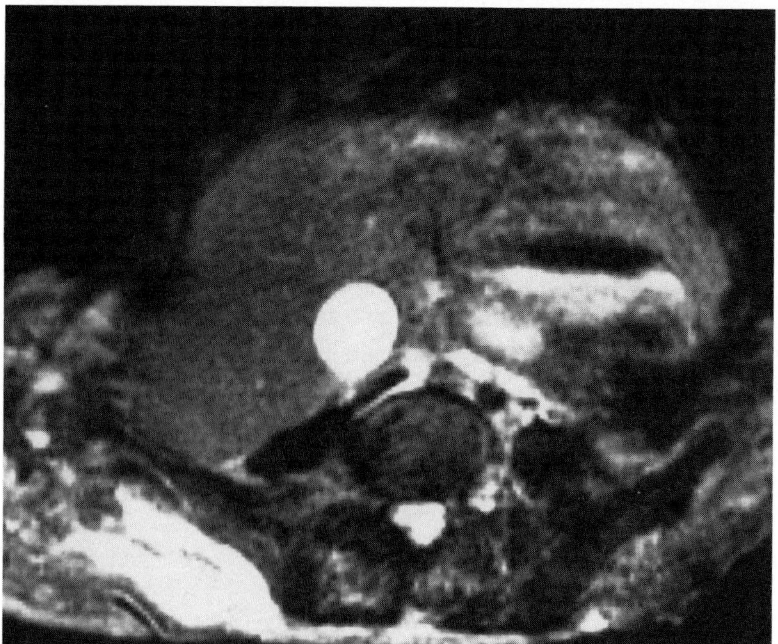

B

FIGURE 5. Axial MRI of the abdomen showing (A) a fluid-fluid level in the gallbladder on a T1-weighted image, with the hyperintense, dependent layer being more concentrated bile, and (B) homogeneous high signal in the gallbladder on a T2-weighted image.

E. Magnetic Resonance Imaging

As with oral cholecystography, MRI primarily images the contents of the normal gallbladder, but lacks the resolution of oral cholecystography. The ability to image in several planes allows clearer depiction of the relationship of the gallbladder to its surrounding structures. The gallbladder wall is barely distinguishable, being isointense with liver on T1- and T2-weighted images.

On T2-weighted images, normal bile may be isointense with or slightly hyperintense to adjacent liver. With longer echo delays (TE 120 to 180 ms) bile has a higher signal intensity, similar to cerebrospinal fluid (CSF). The appearance on T1-weighted images is variable and depends on the water content of the bile. In the immediate postprandial state unconcentrated bile has a high water content and therefore has a low signal on T1-weighted images.[7] With the absorption of water the concentrated bile has a higher signal on T1-weighted images, becoming brighter than adjacent liver. Because concentrated bile is greater in density, a layering effect can be seen with dark, dilute bile above bright, concentrated bile (Figure 5).

REFERENCES

1. **Donald, J. J., Fache, J. S., Buckley, A. R., and Burhenne, H. J.,** Gallbladder contractility: variation in normal subjects, *AJR,* 157, 753, 1991.
2. **Davies, F. and Harding, H. E.,** Pouch of Hartmann, *Lancet,* 1, 193, 1942.
3. **Callen, P. W. and Filly, R. A.,** Ultrasonographic localization of the gallbladder, *Radiology,* 133, 687, 1979.
4. **O'Brien, M. J. and Gottlieb, L. S.,** The liver and biliary tract, in *Pathological Basis of Disease,* Robbins, S. L. and Cotran, R. S., Eds., W. B. Saunders, Philadelphia, 1979.
5. **Berk, R. N., Ferruce, J. T., Jr., and Leopold, G. R.,** *Radiology of the Gallbladder and Bile Ducts, Diagnoses and Intervention.* W. B. Saunders, Philadelphia, 1983.
6. **Marchal, G., Van de Voorde, P., Van Dooren, W., Ponette, E., and Baert, A.,** Ultrasonic appearance of the filled and contracted normal gallbladder, *J. Clin. Ultrasound,* 8, 439, 1980.
7. **Hricak, H., Filly, R. A., Margulis, A. R., Moon, K. L., Crooks, L. E., and Kaufman, L.,** Work in progress: nuclear magnetic resonance imaging of the gallbladder, *Radiology,* 147, 481, 1983.

Chapter 3

EMBRYOLOGY OF THE GALLBLADDER

Abraham H. Dachman and Carson Schneck

The embryologic development of the gallbladder must be discussed in the context of the embryology of the surrounding structures including the biliary tree and liver. A single liver bud or hepatic diverticulum develops at the beginning of embryonic week 4. It forms as an endodermal outgrowth from the ventral aspect of the caudal portion of the foregut. This is the site where the descending portion of the duodenum will develop. This single hepatic diverticulum will ultimately develop into the liver, gallbladder, biliary tree, and ventral portion of the pancreas[1–4] (Figure 1A).

The liver primordium is formed by proliferation of the cephalic portion of the hepatic diverticulum as it invades the septum transversum. Cellular proliferation and differentiation occurs to form liver cells and the epithelial lining of the intrahepatic biliary tree. The initial pattern of cellular proliferation during the formation of the primordial hepatic ducts is one of a diffuse plexus which is much more extensive than that seen in the mature fetus. Many of these ducts will ultimately involute with the remaining ducts forming the definitive hepatic duct pattern. A relatively narrow channel persists as a connection between the liver primordium and the foregut. This persistent channel will give rise to the epithelial lining of the remainder of the extrahepatic biliary tree.

The gallbladder and cystic duct develop as ventral extensions from this channel connecting the liver primordium to the developing duodenum (Figure 1B). This occurs at approximately embryonic week 4. At the same time, a ventral pancreatic primordium develops as an outpouching off the narrow extrahepatic biliary channel near the duodenum. When the ventral pancreatic primordium has appeared sometime in the beginning of embryonic week 5, all the early precursors of hepatobiliary anatomy are present: gallbladder, cystic duct, hepatic ducts, common bile duct, ventral pancreas. All these structures are contained within the ventral mesentery of the duodenum. In the next growth phase during week 5 of life, the extrahepatic portion of the biliary tree elongates, although its diameter remains relatively constant. This is a stage of rapid elongation in which epithelial proliferation causes the entire extrahepatic biliary system to become a solid core of cells.

Further development in rotation of structures in this area is thought to be due to a differential growth of the wall of the duodenum. Sometime at the end of embryonic week 5 this differential growth causes a change in the position of both the hepatic and ventral pancreatic diverticula. Although originally located ventrally, the elongation and growth of the duodenum

0-8493-4788-2/94/$0.00+$.50

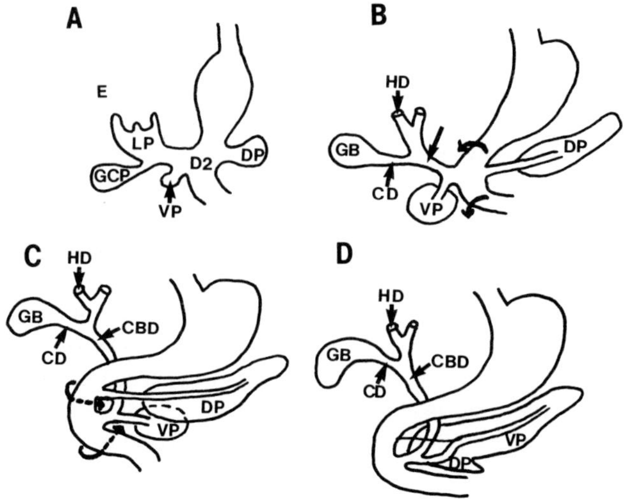

FIGURE 1. Embryological development of the gallbladder and biliary tract. (A) is a lateral view of the early development of the liver primordium (LP), gallbladder-cystic duct primordium (GCP), ventral pancreas (VP), and dorsal pancreas (DP) from the second part of the duodenum (D2) in the 4-week embryo. (B) is a lateral view of the 5-week embryo showing differentiation of the hepatic ducts (HD), gallbladder (GB), cystic duct (CD), and common bile duct (CBD) at their solid cell stage. (C) is a lateral view of an early 6-week embryo demonstrating how the proliferation of the epithelium of the left wall of the duodenum causes the common bile duct and main pancreatic ducts to migrate into the dorsal mesentery. (D) is an anterior view of the late 6-week embryo showing the relationships after the duodenal loop has rotated to the right to form a fusion fascia with the retroperitoneum. (From Friedman, A. C. and Dachman, A., *Radiology of the Liver, Biliary Tract and Pancreas,* Mosby Year Book, St. Louis, 1993. With permission.)

causes a shift of the hepatic and ventral pancreatic diverticula to a dorsal location just below the origin of the dorsal pancreatic primordium (Figure 1C). This differential growth of the duodenum, with greater epithelial proliferation of the left aspect of the duodenum, accounts for the movement of the common bile duct and main pancreatic duct to the dorsal aspect of the duodenum. Simultaneously, there is a 90° rotation of the duodenal loop to the right. This explains why the common bile duct and main pancreatic duct open on the posterior medial aspect of the descending portion of the duodenum.

As the duodenum grows in length it forms a ventrally directed loop. The apex of this duodenal loop marks the point of junction between the foregut and the midgut. At a point just cranial to this foregut-midgut junction is the site of the hepatic diverticulum. While the stomach (which is posteriorly directed) rotates to the left, the inferiorly directed duodenal loop rotates to the right, causing the right side of the second, third, and fourth parts of the duodenum and the dorsal mesentery to push against the parietal peritoneum.

Subsequently, a fusion of the opposed peritoneal membranes forms a fusion fascia (Figure 1D). By this time, both the ventral pancreatic primordium and the lower portion of the common bile duct have rotated dorsally into the dorsal mesentery to join the dorsal pancreatic primordium. The lower part of the common bile duct and the ventral pancreatic primordium will also form a fusion fascia over the retroperitoneal organs (aorta, inferior vena cava, kidneys, and adrenal glands). Thus, the duodenum, pancreas, and lower common bile duct, although originally developing within mesenteries, are said to become secondarily retroperitoneal. The retroperitoneal organs, along with the fusion fascia that develops between the organs as described above, contribute to the formation of the anterior layer of Gerota's fascia.

The rotation of the duodenal loop to the right causes the more superior or proximal part of the common bile duct to lie posterior to the first part of the duodenum. The infraduodenal or intrapancreatic portion of the common bile duct becomes retroperitoneal. Because the first part of the duodenum retains its ventral and dorsal mesenteries, the retroduodenal part of the common bile duct is peritonealized. The portion of the common bile duct that is supraduodenal ascends in that portion of the ventral mesentery that ultimately becomes the hepatoduodenal ligament (Figure 1D). At the level of the epiploic foramen it lies in the anterior wall of the foramen in juxtaposition to the developing portal vein and proper hepatic artery. Thus, the developing cystic duct and common hepatic ducts were also situated in this portion of the ventral mesentery. When the duodenal loop rotates to the right, the ventral mesentery becomes reoriented into a coronal plane from its original sagittal orientation.

At around the sixth embryonic week the developing extrahepatic biliary tree becomes organized. Slowly, reestablishment of the lumen of the extrahepatic biliary tree occurs via a process of recanalization which progresses in a proximal fashion. At about the seventh week, the lumen reaches the cystic duct, but the gallbladder is still a solid mass of cells until week 12 (Figure 2).

If this process of recanalization proceeds abnormally and there is failure of recanalization involving either the bile ducts or gallbladder, various forms of atresia may result. During the recanalization process it is possible for two or more lumina to coexist temporally within a duct. While these eventually coalesce to form a single lumen, they may fail to coalesce, explaining some duplication anomalies.

Small, rudimentary accessory hepatic ducts exist that open into the hepatic or cystic ducts. During development, most of these involute. During the ninth week, the muscular parts of the gallbladder develop from the mesenchymal cells surrounding the gallbladder epithelial primordium. There is a progressive development of the muscular coats toward the duodenum.

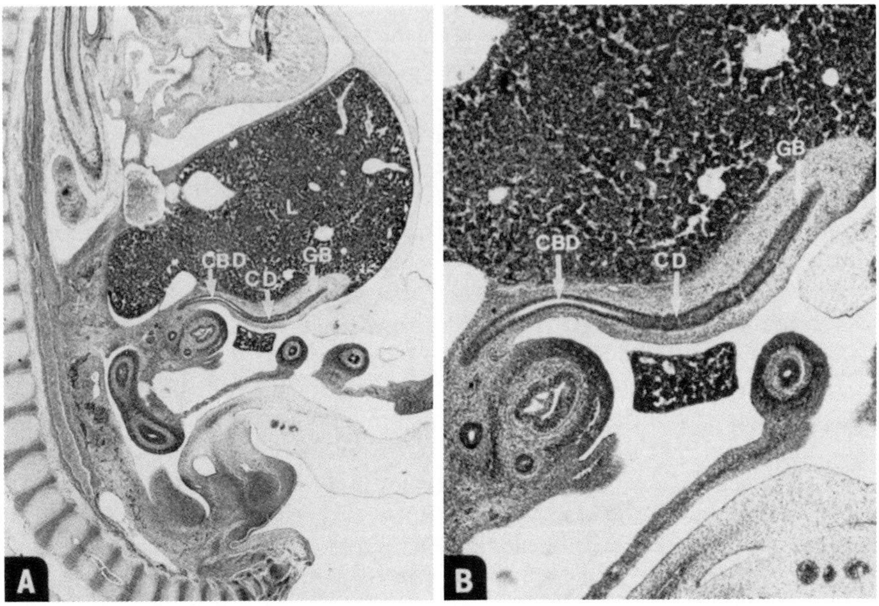

FIGURE 2. Micrograph of the developing biliary system. (A) is a sagittal section through the abdomen of a 7-week embryo demonstrating the gallbladder (GB), cystic duct (CD), and common bile duct (CBD) lying on the visceral surface of the liver (L) just superior to the duodenum (D). (B) is a magnified view of (A) demonstrating the recanalization of the common bile duct while the gallbladder and cystic duct are still a solid mass of cells. (From Friedman, A. C. and Dachman, A., *Radiology of the Liver, Biliary Tract and Pancreas*, Mosby Year Book, St. Louis, 1993. With permission.)

While specific congenital abnormalities are discussed in detail later in this volume, specific embryologic explanations for some of these anomalies are presented here.

As described above, the usual explanation for various forms of extrahepatic biliary atresia is that of failure of recanalization of the solid epithelial cords which develop during embryonic week 5. Normally, recanalization occurs between weeks 6 and 12. Thus, the abnormality that leads to extrahepatic biliary atresia probably occurs between weeks 6 and 12. It therefore makes sense that between 10 and 30% of patients with biliary atresia may have associated anomalies that may be explained by organs that develop concurrently. Coexistent abnormalities such as annular pancreas, malrotation, duodenal atresia, imperforate anus, portal and inferior vena cava anomalies, polysplenia, congenital heart disease, and urinary tract anomalies may be explained in this fashion.[6–8] There may be evidence of reovirus type 3 infection implicated as a possible cause of biliary atresia in infants.[9]

It is interesting that gallbladder agenesis may occur in association with extrahepatic biliary atresia. This probably represents a similar mechanism of failure of recanalization. However, gallbladder agenesis, although rare, may occur in association with a normal biliary tree. Up to one sixth of patients with extrahepatic biliary atresia also have gallbladder agenesis.[10] When gallbladder agenesis occurs the cystic duct is usually absent as well. This implies that there is complete failure of development of the gallbladder-cystic duct bud in the 5-week embryo. If there is a vestigial or hypoplastic gallbladder or a dilated cystic duct stump without a gallbladder this probably represents abnormal development of the gallbladder-cystic duct primordium.[3]

In order to explain abnormalities of gallbladder location, recall that during the second fetal month the liver grows rapidly. This causes the liver to bulge down, out of the septum transversum, into the abdominal cavity. It is thought that the gallbladder then becomes imbedded within the liver. Various rates of growth may explain the common positional anomalies of the gallbladder: intrahepatic, retrohepatic, left-sided, and ptotic (hanging) gallbladder. The retrohepatic gallbladder is thought to result from an abnormal posterior migration of the gallbladder-cystic duct bud. When a left-sided gallbladder occurs as a rare, solitary anomaly (without situs inversus), the gallbladder will lie on the undersurface of the left lobe of the liver to the left of the falciform ligament.[10] The left-sided gallbladder may have a cystic duct, arising in the usual position, but angling sharply to the left. This sharp turn to the left suggests an abnormal migration of a normally arising gallbladder-cystic duct bud. A left-sided gallbladder may also arise from the left side of either the left hepatic duct or the junction of the common hepatic and common bile ducts, indicating an abnormal left-sided origin of the gallbladder-cystic duct bud. The ptotic gallbladder may occur as an acquired or a congenital condition. When it is congenital (and found in a young patient) it may represent a failure of the gallbladder-cystic duct bud to reach the liver, resulting in retention of some or all of the original mesenteric origin.

In week 12, when the gallbladder becomes hollow by vacuolization, incomplete vacuolization may result in a septation within the gallbladder. If complete septation exists, this represents a true duplication of the gallbladder. In fact, varying degrees of duplication of the gallbladder may occur. An external duplication may involve only the fundus or a varying amount of the body to the level of the neck (Figure 3A to C). A mild form of duplication may involve internal longitudinal septation, which completely separates the gallbladder into two chambers but without external evidence of duplication[3,10,11] (Figure 3A). Partial duplications are formed by a single gallbladder-cystic duct bud, which bifurcates at some point after it begins to grow. This may result in partial duplication of the cystic duct along its course, yet a single cystic duct may open into the common bile

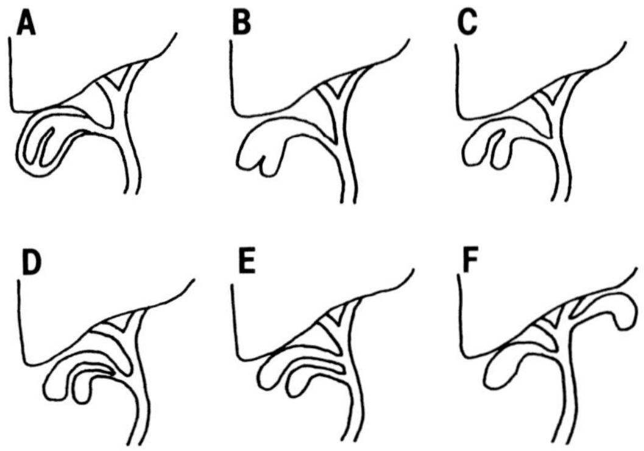

FIGURE 3. Gallbladder duplication. (A) Septate gallbladder. (B) Fundic duplication. (C) Body duplication. (D) Y-shaped gallbladder. (E) Complete duplication. (F) Bilateral gallbladders. (From Friedman, A. C. and Dachman, A., *Radiology of the Liver, Biliary Tract and Pancreas*, Mosby Year Book, St. Louis, 1993. With permission.)

duct (Figure 3D). Complete duplications involving both the gallbladder and the cystic duct, with two complete cystic duct openings into the biliary system, may also exist. In this case, the two gallbladders commonly lie side by side and the cystic ducts may join the common hepatic or right hepatic duct (Figure 3E). Rarely, the dual gallbladders may lie on opposite sides of the common hepatic duct in which case the left-sided gallbladder may have its cystic duct opening into the left hepatic duct (Figure 3F). A complete duplication of both gallbladder and cystic duct implies that 2 gallbladder-cystic duct outpouchings developed in the 5-week embryo.

An embryonic bend in the terminal part of the gallbladder-cystic duct outgrowth may account for deformities such as Phrygian cap, hourglass gallbladder, Hartmann's pouch, and diverticula. Not all these abnormalities are necessarily congenital in origin. For example, Hartmann's pouch is also thought to form as an acquired dilation of the infundibulum in response to chronic obstruction.[3] Gallbladder diverticula may likewise be acquired, but in cases such as fundic diverticula, may represent an arrest of development of the tip of the gallbladder-cystic bud.[3]

Anomalies of the common bile duct may accompany anomalies of the gallbladder, however, a detailed discussion of the embryology of these abnormalities is beyond the scope of this volume.

REFERENCES

1. **Sadler, T. W.,** *Langman's Medical Embryology*, 5th ed., Williams & Wilkins, Baltimore, 1985, 230.
2. **Moore, K. L.,** *The Developing Human*, 3rd ed., W. B. Saunders, Philadelphia, 1972, 233.
3. **Gray, S. W. and Skandalakis, J. E.,** *Embryology for Surgeons*, 1st ed., W. B. Saunders, Philadelphia, 1972, 224.
4. **Netter, F. H. and Oppenheimer, E.,** *Liver, Biliary Tract and Pancreas*, Ciba collection of medical illustrations, Digestive system, Ciba, New Jersey, 2, 1964, 23.
5. **Shim, W. K. T., Kasai, M., and Spence, M. A.,** Racial influence on the incidence of biliary atresia, *Prog. Pediatr. Surg.*, 6, 53, 1974.
6. **Guzzetta, P. C., Anderson, K. D., Altman, R. P., Newman, K. D., Eichelberger, K. R., and Randolph, J. R.,** Pediatric surgery, in *Principles of Surgery*, Vol. 2, 5th ed., Schwartz, S. L., Shives, G. T., and Spencer, F. C., Eds., McGraw-Hill, New York, 1989, 1687.
7. **Lilly, J. R.,** Biliary atresia: the jaundiced infant, in *Pediatric Surgery*, 4th ed., Welch, K. J., Randolph, J. G., Ravitch, M. M., O'Neill, J. A., and Row, M. I., Eds., Year Book Medical Publishers, Chicago, 1986, 1047.
8. **Grossfeld, J. L.,** Pediatric surgery, *Textbook of Surgery*, 14th ed., Sabistan, D. C., Ed., W. B. Saunders, Philadelphia, 1991, 1170.
9. **Morecki, R., Slaser, J., Cho, S., Balistreri, W. F., and Horwitz, M. S.,** Biliary atresia and reovirus type 3 infection, *N. Engl. J. Med.*, 307, 481, 1982.
10. **Gross, R. E.,** Congenital anomalies of the gallbladder, *Arch. Surg.*, 32, 131, 1936.
11. **Hollinshead, W. H.,** The thorax, abdomen and pelvis, in *Anatomy for Surgeons*, Vol. 2, 2nd ed., Harper & Row, New York, 1971, 314.

Chapter 4

THE FETAL GALLBLADDER

Jon W. Meilstrup, Kenneth D. Hopper, and Claudia J. Kasales

During fetal development the gallbladder is a solid structure through week 12 of gestation.[1,2] As a result, it is not visualized on fetal sonography before the second trimester of pregnancy. By gestational week 20, however, the gallbladder closely resembles its pediatric counterpart, and can be identified in up to 65% of fetuses. It appears as a fluid-filled structure to the right of the umbilical vein. The neck is typically narrower than the fundus, resulting in a conical or ovoid gallbladder appearance (Figure 1). Its shape and typical location help to distinguish the gallbladder from the umbilical vein, although occasionally color Doppler imaging may be necessary to aid in differentiating these two structures.[1,3–6]

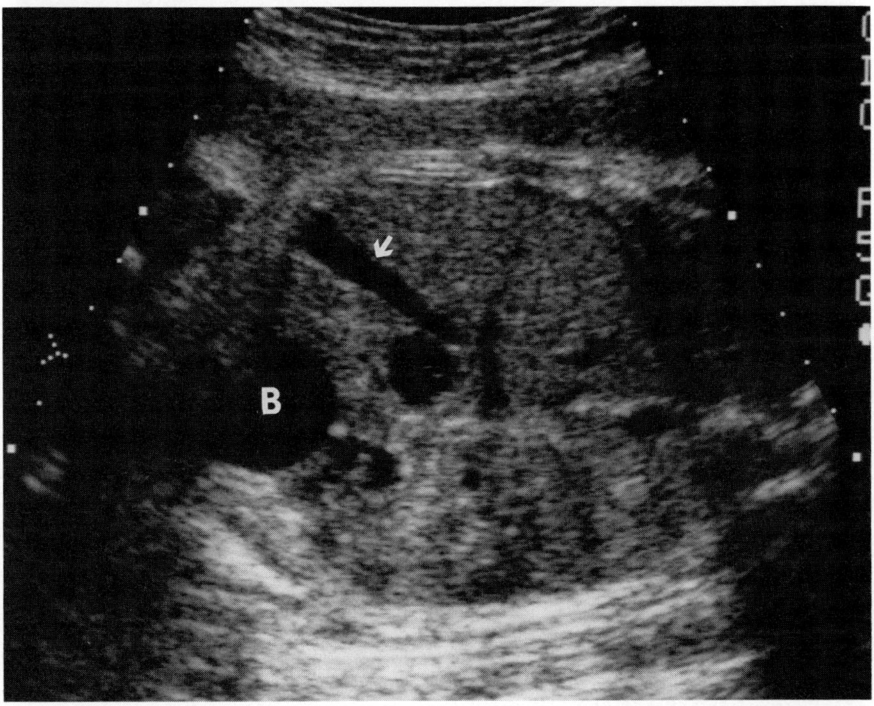

FIGURE 1. Oblique-transverse view through a fetal abdomen shows a normal gallbladder (arrow). The insonation angle is steep in order to include the entire gallbladder, which results in visualization of the urinary bladder (B) on the same image.

0–8493–4788–2/94/$0.00+$.50

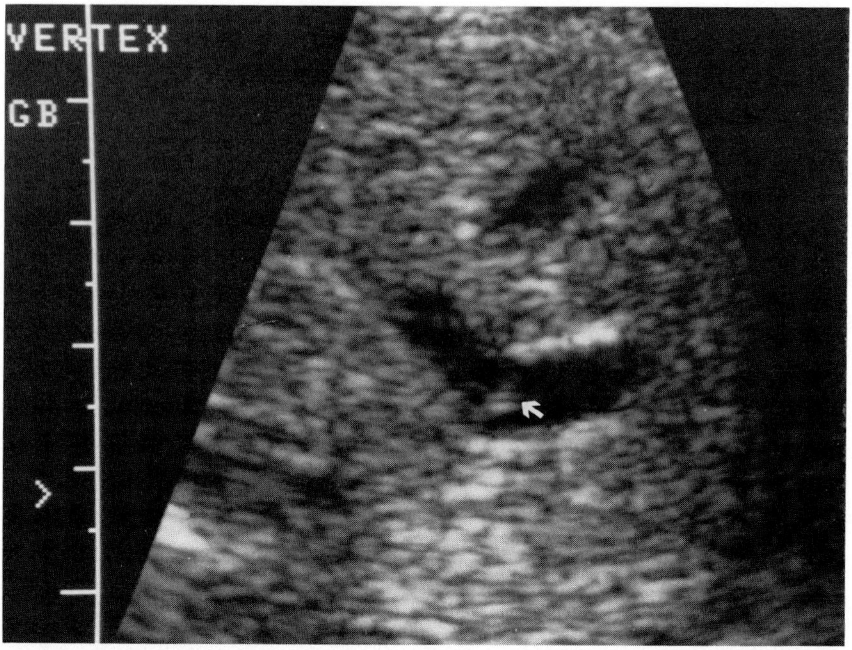

FIGURE 2. Magnified view of a fetal gallbladder shows a fold or septation (arrow).

Dilation of the fetal gallbladder can be normal and should not be diagnosed as pathologic with only one ultrasound examination. Comparison with normal fetal measurements of length, width, and area (available after 20 weeks' gestational age)[1] may be helpful in the evaluation of such dilation. However, administration of a fatty meal to the fasting mother generally is not useful because the fetal gallbladder has not been shown to have an active physiologic role *in utero*.[6–8]

With improvement in ultrasound imaging resolution, several gallbladder anomalies have been described on prenatal ultrasound examination, including gallbladder septation[7] (Figure 2), folds (Figure 3), and duplication.[9] Ectopic fetal gallbladder locations should be considered on prenatal examinations when a cystic, ovoid structure is present within the abdomen and a normally located gallbladder is not evident.

While nonvisualization of the gallbladder is not uncommon during prenatal sonography, repeated studies without gallbladder visualization may indicate agenesis, especially if associated with biliary atresia, polysplenia, or cardiac anomalies.[4]

Viscous, echogenic bile, or sludge can be seen occasionally within the fetal gallbladder, and has been associated with fetal hepatitis,[4] as well as maternal cholelithiasis and cholestasis.[10] More commonly, however, it is found in normal fetuses. In one series of 26 third-trimester sonograms

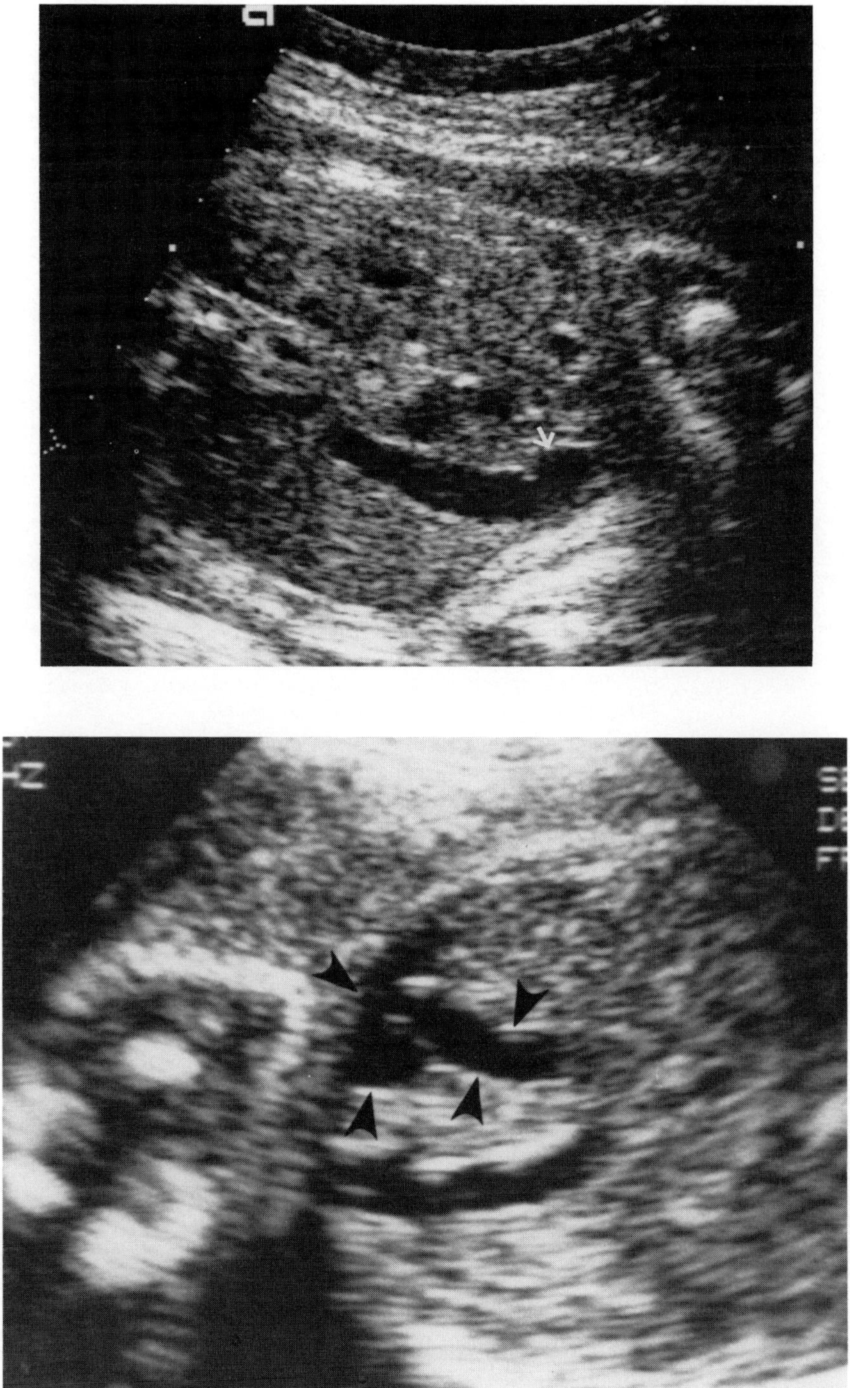

FIGURE 3. (A) Fetal Phrygian cap (arrow). (B) Fetal gallbladder (arrowheads) with Phrygian cap showing greater fundal folding than A. (Part B is courtesy of Dr. Michael Manco-Johnson, University of Colorado.)

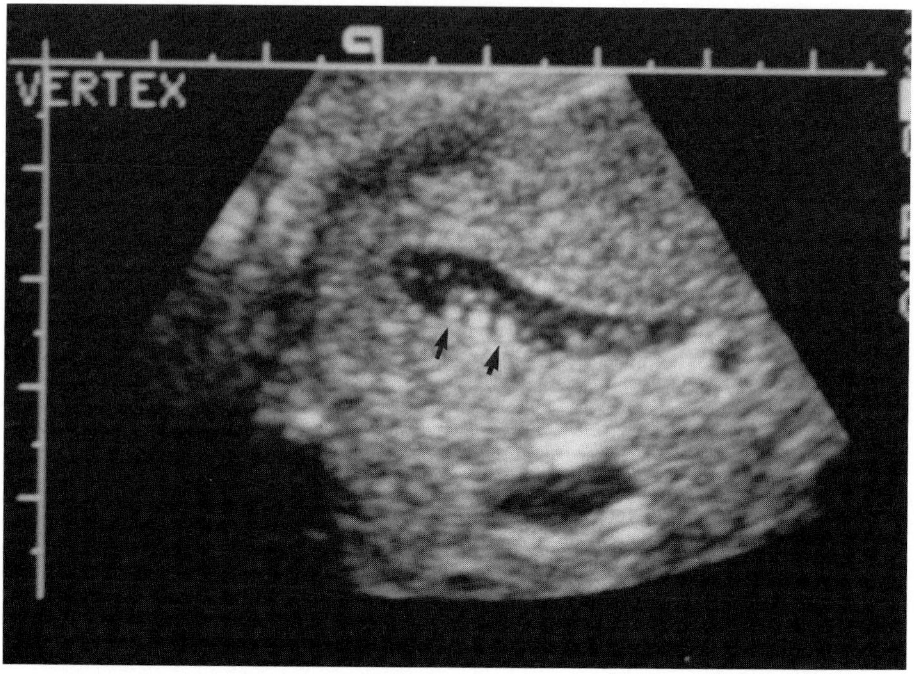

FIGURE 4. Fetal gallstones (arrows) and sludge.

showing sludge within the fetal gallbladder, neither common etiology nor clinical sequelae were found.[11] Fetal sludge has been noted to resolve on sequential sonograms, but is less likely to occur if the bile attenuates the ultrasound beam, causing distal shadowing. Because its natural history is poorly understood, a postnatal sonogram should be performed on any fetus with echogenic bile.[11]

Fetal gallstones have been reported on prenatal ultrasound examination[12–14] (Figure 4). Like gallstones in children or adults, they are mobile and echogenic; however, they may not cast acoustic shadows. No specific abnormality has been consistently associated with fetal gallstones. However, hemolytic anemias should be considered because they are the most frequent cause of gallstones in the pediatric age group.[14,15] One fetus with reported gallstones later demonstrated mild spherocytosis as a neonate,[12] but most affected fetuses are normal at birth. A possible association with maternal narcotic use also has been suggested.[16] Because fetal gallstones often resolve spontaneously, their clinical significance is uncertain.[12,13,15–17] Therefore, a conservative approach to such a fetus is generally recommended, including postnatal ultrasound evaluation.[4,13]

Cystohepatic ducts are fetal communications between the gallbladder and the intrahepatic biliary ducts. While they have been described in neonates, they are usually not present in the adult, and their radiographic or ultrasonographic appearance has not been described.[18] However, remnants of these ducts (known as the ducts or crypts of Luschka)[19] can be identified in 10 to 15% of adult gallbladders at autopsy. Their presence has no known clinical significance.

Though little is known about the fetal gallbladder, familiarity with anomalies of position, size, and shape can be helpful in the evaluation of cystic fetal abdominal masses. Fetal sludge and gallstones are rarely seen, but generally can be followed conservatively with postnatal sonography. Clinical correlation with possible hemolytic disease should be considered in these infants.

REFERENCES

1. **Hata, K., Showa, A., Hata, T., Murao, F., and Kitao, M.,** Ultrasonographic identification of the human fetal gallbladder in utero, *Gynecol. Obstet. Invest.*, 23, 79, 1987.
2. **Gray, S. W. and Skandalakis, J. E.,** *Embryology for Surgeons,* W. B. Saunders, Philadelphia, 1972, 229.
3. **Comstock, C. H. and Kirk, J. S.,** The fetal chest and abdomen, in *Diagnostic Ultrasound,* Vol. 2, Rumack, C., Wilson, S. R., and Charboneau, J. W., Eds., Mosby Year Book, St. Louis, 1991, chap. 37.
4. **Nyberg, D. A.,** Intra-abdominal abnormalities, in *Diagnostic Ultrasound of Fetal Anomalies: Text and Atlas,* Nyberg, D. A., Mahony, B. S., and Pretorius, D. H., Eds., Year Book Medical Publishers, Chicago, 1990, chap. 10.
5. **Romero, R., Pilu, G., Jeanty, P., Ghidini, A., and Hobbins, J. C.,** in *Prenatal Diagnosis of Congenital Anomalies,* Appleton and Lange, Norwalk, CT, 1988, 234.
6. **Hertzberg, B. S. and Bowie, J. D.,** Sonographic evaluation of abnormalities of the fetal gastrointestinal tract, in *The Principles and Practice of Ultrasonography in Obstetrics and Gynecology,* 4th ed., Fleischer, A. C., Romero, R., Manning, F. A., Jeanty, P., and James, Jr., A. E., Eds., Appleton and Lange, Norwalk, CT, 1991, 245.
7. **Sherer, D. M., Hearn-Stebbins, B., Manuli, M. G., and Abramowicz, J. S.,** Gallbladder, septation, *Fetus,* 2(6), 7516 **(3)**, 1992.
8. **Jouppila, P., Heikkinen, J., and Kerkinen, P.,** Contractility of maternal and fetal gallbladder: an ultrasonic study, *J. Clin. Ultrasound,* 13, 461, 1985.
9. **Sutter, W. B. and Jeanty, P.,** Gallbladder, duplication, *Fetus,* 1(3), 7516 **(1)**, 1991.
10. **Penzias, A. S. and Treisman, O.,** Vitamin K-dependent clotting factor deficiency in pregnancy, *Obstet. Gynecol.,* 72, 452, 1988.
11. **Brown, D. L., Teele, R. L., Doubilet, P. I. M., DiSalvo, D. N., Benson, C. B., and Van Alstyne, G. R.,** Echogenic material in the fetal gallbladder: sonographic and clinical observations, *Radiology,* 182, 73, 1992.
12. **Beretsky, I. and Lankin, D. H.,** Diagnosis of fetal cholelithiasis using real-time high-resolution imaging employing digital detection, *J. Ultrasound Med.,* 2, 381, 1983.

13. **Klingensmith, W. C. and Cioffi-Ragan, D. T.,** Fetal gallstones, *Radiology*, 167, 143, 1988.
14. **Mukuno, D. H., Lee, T. G., Harnsberger, H. R., and Cubberly, D. A.,** Sonography of the fetal gastrointestinal system, *Semin. Ultrasound CT MR*, 5, 194, 1984.
15. **Henschke, C. I. and Teele, R. L.,** Cholelithiasis in children: recent observations, *J. Ultrasound Med.*, 2, 481, 1983.
16. **Devonald, K. J., Ellwood, D. A., and Colditz, P. B.,** The variable appearances of fetal gallstones, *J. Ultrasound Med.*, 11, 579, 1992.
17. **Keller, M. S., Markle, B. M., Laffey, P. A., Chawla, H. S., Jacir, N., and Frank, J. L.,** Spontaneous resolution of cholelithiasis in infants, *Radiology*, 157, 345, 1985.
18. **Hatfield, P. M. and Wise, R. E.,** Anatomic variation in the gallbladder and bile ducts, *Semin. Roentgenol.*, 11, 157, 1976.
19. **Robertson, H. E. and Ferguson, W. J.,** The diverticula (Luschka's crypts) of the gallbladder, *Arch. Pathol.*, 40, 312, 1945.

Chapter 5

VARIATIONS OF LOCATION

Jon W. Meilstrup and Kenneth D. Hopper

TABLE OF CONTENTS

0–8493–4788–2/94/$0.00+$.50

I. INTRODUCTION

While the gallbladder is usually located in the right upper quadrant, it can be found virtually anywhere in the abdomen and pelvis. Although anomalous positions of the gallbladder are uncommon, their occurrence, if not appreciated, can cause potentially serious misdiagnoses.[1,2] When the gallbladder is not visualized in its normal location, a careful search should be made to exclude an ectopic location, including the left abdomen, because a diseased left-sided gallbladder can refer symptoms to the right upper quadrant or mid-epigastric regions.[3]

II. LEFT UPPER QUADRANT[4–14]

When the gallbladder is seen in the left abdomen, it is usually associated with situs inversus (Figure 1). It is rare to see an isolated left-sided gallbladder. Other causes of a left-sided gallbladder include a ''floating'' gallbladder, herniation of the gallbladder into the lesser sac, or as a finding associated with intestinal malrotation.[11] A duplicated gallbladder can even have a normally located right gallbladder with the accompanying second gallbladder on the left side.[13]

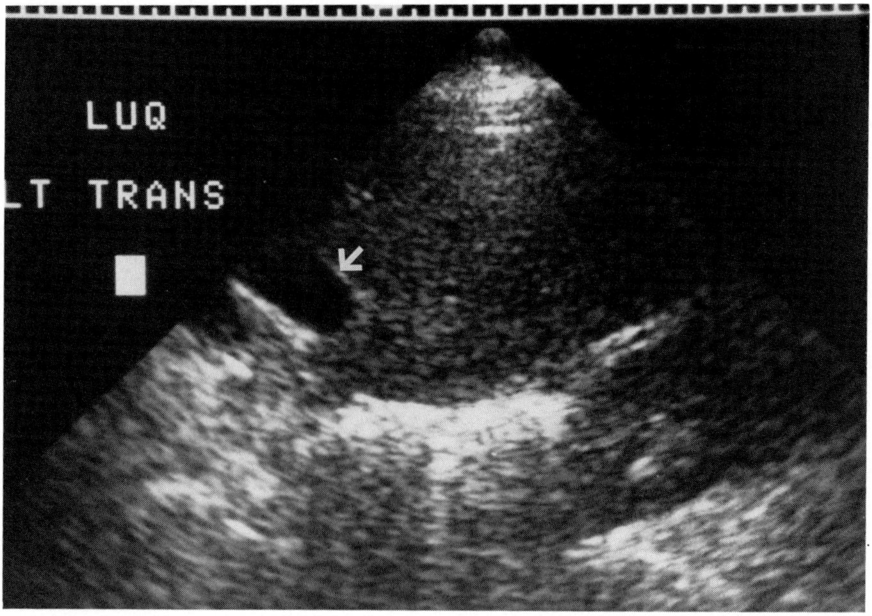

FIGURE 1. Transverse sonogram shows the gallbladder (arrow) in the left upper quadrant of the abdomen, medial to a left-sided liver in a patient with situs inversus. (From Meilstrup, J. W., Hopper, K. D., and Thieme, G. A., *AJR*, 157, 1205, 1991. With permission.)

It has been theorized that a left-sided gallbladder occurs when the embryological gallbladder bud off the hepatic diverticulum migrates toward the left rather than the right. Another possible cause of a left-sided gallbladder is the development of a separate gallbladder bud directly from the left hepatic duct, with the normal right gallbladder not developing.[7]

III. INTRAHEPATIC

The intrahepatic gallbladder lies within the substance of the liver, such that little or none of the gallbladder is seen on the external hepatic surface.[15] The portion of the gallbladder imbedded in the liver is variable; occasionally, surgeons and pathologists have noted that only a small part of an intrahepatic gallbladder neck or a tip of the fundus may protrude from the liver.[16] In fact, an intrahepatic gallbladder may be difficult or impossible to visualize at surgery.[15] This type of gallbladder probably results from a developmental anomaly[15] or "congenital arrest"[7] which prevents the gallbladder from changing from its intrahepatic position in the second month of gestation to its normal superficial location.[15]

The intrahepatic gallbladder is readily imaged, especially with sonography and computed tomography (CT) (Figures 2, 3, and Figure 14C, Chapter 9). The gallbladder's position, as well as the appearance of surrounding liver parenchyma, suggests the diagnosis. On scintigraphy, an intrahepatic gallbladder may appear as a focal liver lesion or mimic a choledochal cyst.[2,17,18]

An intrahepatic gallbladder frequently has impaired function because it does not empty completely. As a result, a high percentage of patients develop gallstones, probably related to this bile stasis.[15] Empyema in an intrahepatic gallbladder also has been reported.[19]

IV. TRANSVERSE

Occasionally a horizontal gallbladder position underneath the right lobe of the liver is seen (Figure 4). This horizontal orientation may originate during fetal development due to malrotation or migration of the gallbladder bud.[7,16]

V. RETROPLACED OR RETROPOSITIONED

The gallbladder can lie posterior and inferior to the right hepatic lobe, with the origin of the cystic duct remaining normal.[7] This variant is readily detected on CT, sonography (Figures 5 and 6), and scintigraphy.[20] Retroposition of the gallbladder, particularly if retroperitoneal, can cause confusing symptoms when the gallbladder is diseased, presenting with costovertebral angle tenderness rather than the usual right upper quadrant pain. As with other ectopic locations, such preoperative knowledge is critical for appropriate surgical approach and treatment.[1]

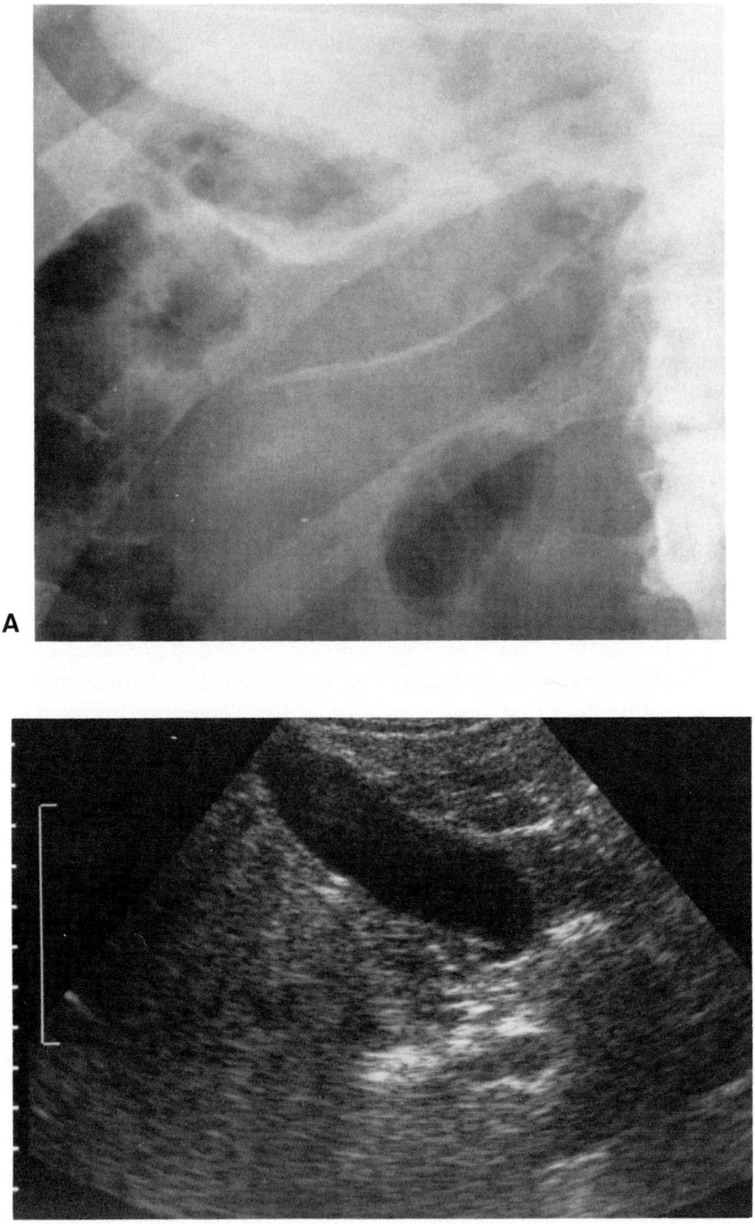

A

B

FIGURE 2. Four different patients with intrahepatic gallbladder: (A) oral cholecystography shows gallbladder in high, transverse position; (B) longitudinal sonogram of gallbladder, with fundus oriented toward head of patient inside the liver substance; (C) CT showing fat and hepatic parenchyma around the gallbladder in the gallbladder fossa; (D) intrahepatic gallbladder on scintigraphy.

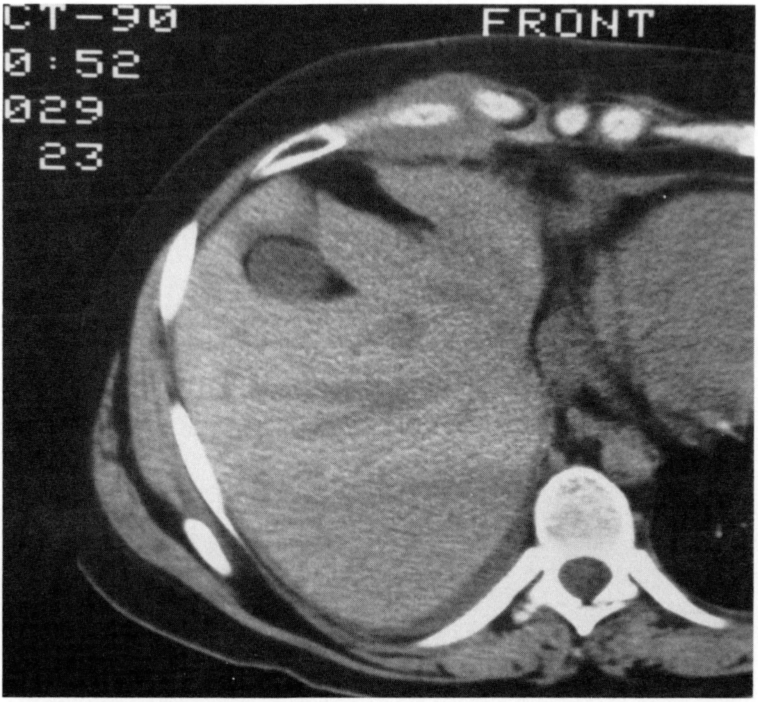

C

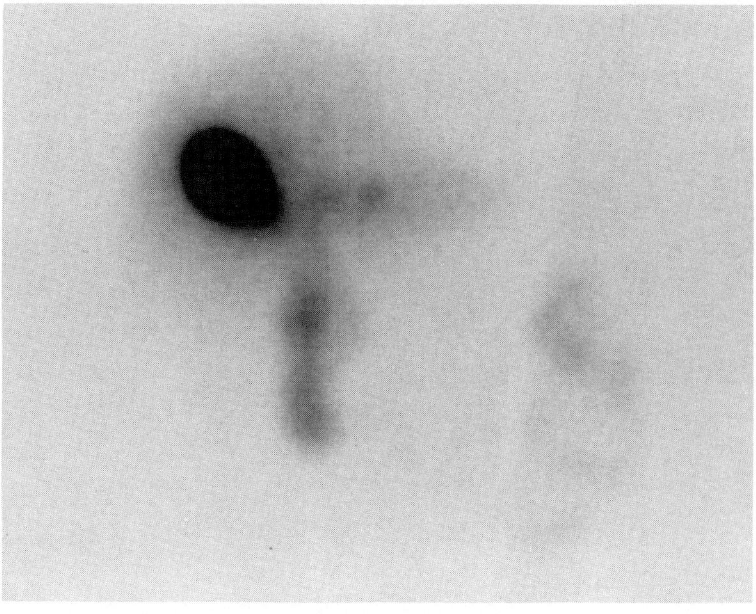

D

FIGURE 2. *Continued.*

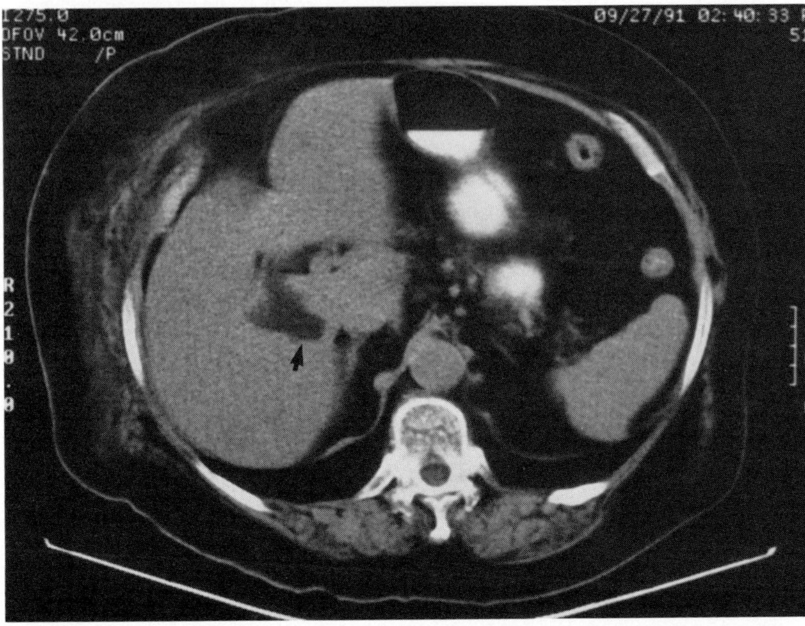

FIGURE 3. CT image of a posterior right intrahepatic gallbladder (arrow), an unusual variation of the intrahepatic gallbladder.

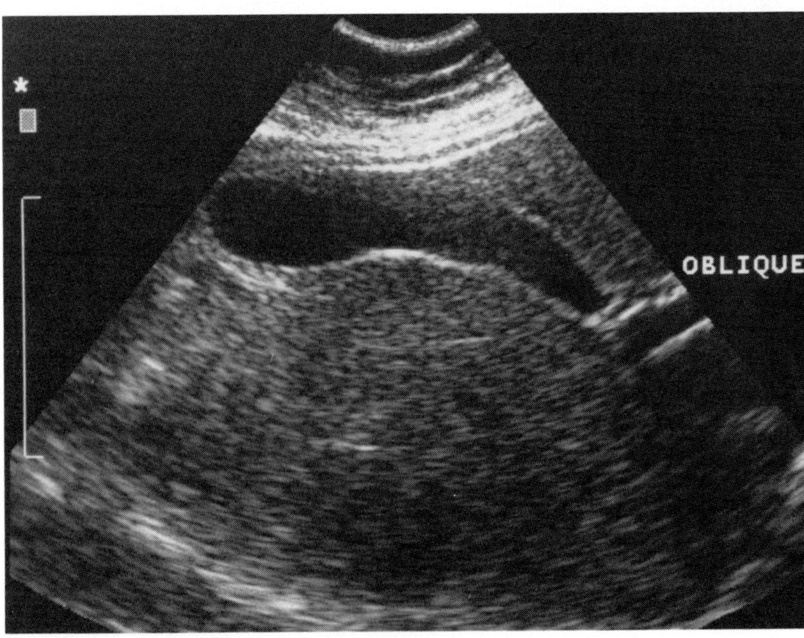

FIGURE 4. Transverse sonogram with slight obliquity shows horizontal orientation of the gallbladder.

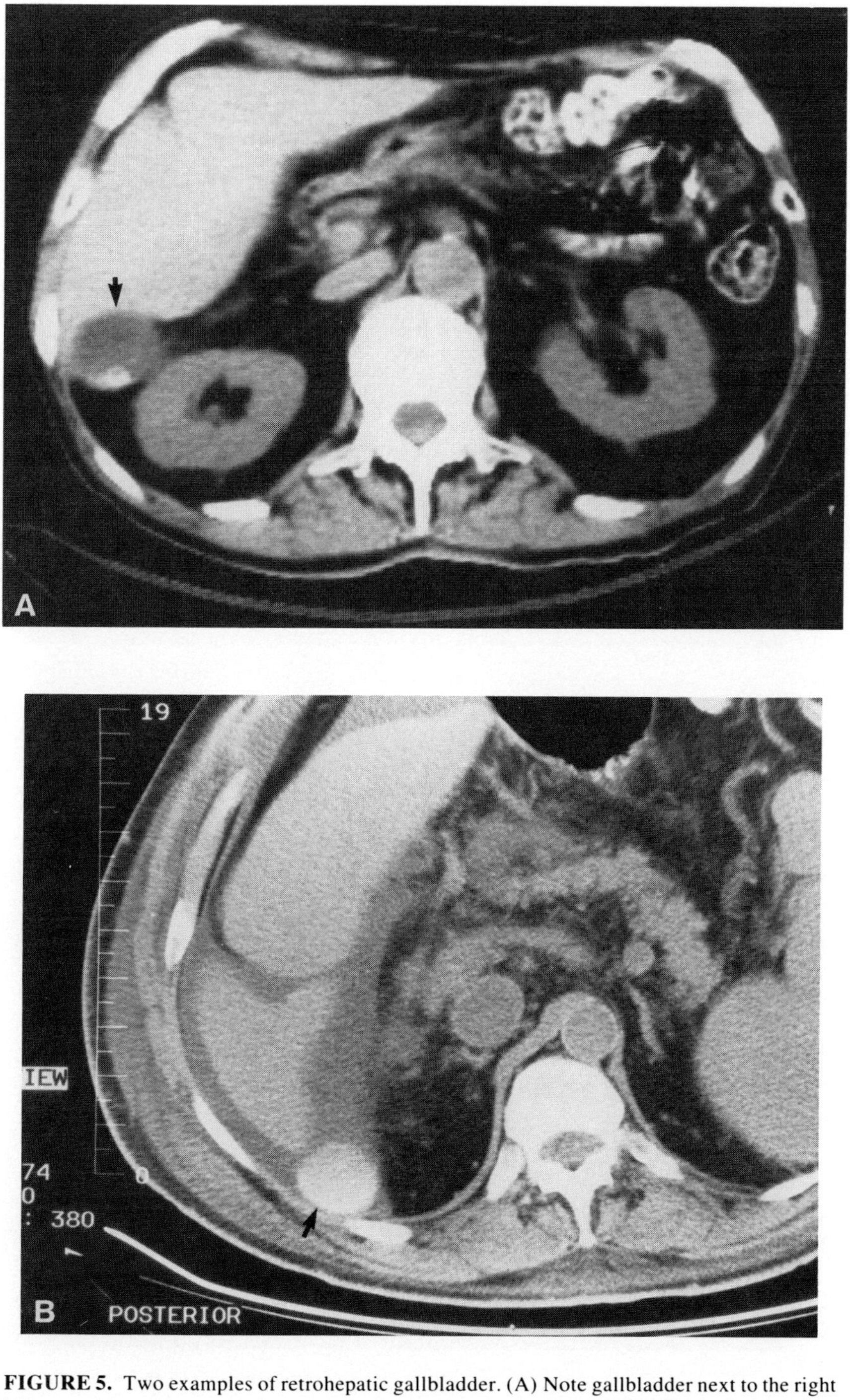

FIGURE 5. Two examples of retrohepatic gallbladder. (A) Note gallbladder next to the right kidney, with gallstone. (B) Dense appearance of retrohepatic gallbladder (arrow) is due to milk of calcium bile. Note hypoplasia of right hepatic lobe, surrounded by ascites.

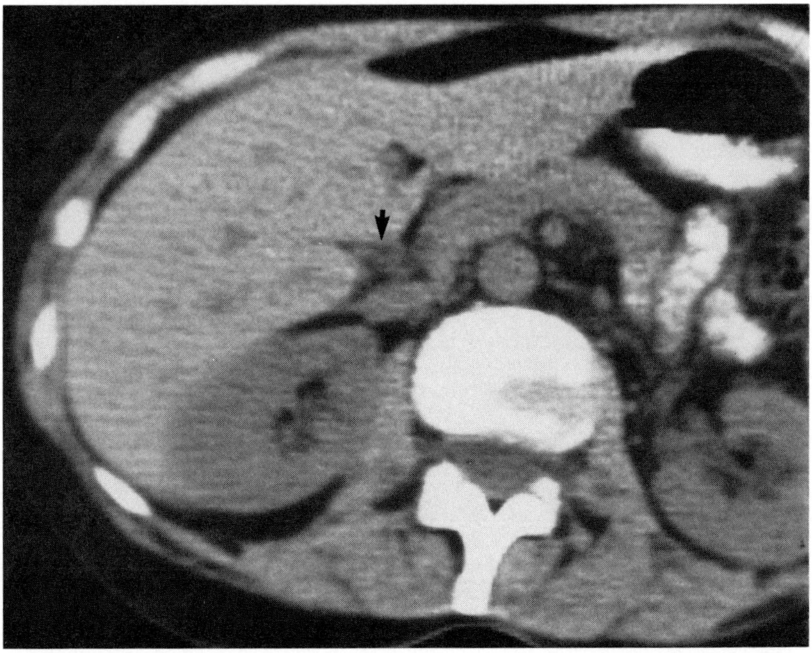

A

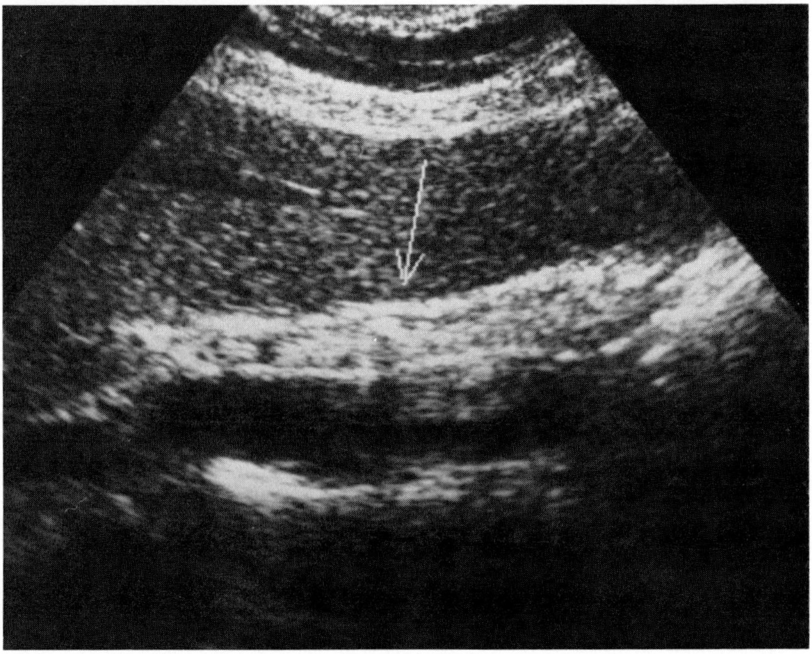

B

FIGURE 6. Images from a 58-year-old female with a contracted retrohepatic gallbladder (arrow) seen on (A) CT, (B) longitudinal sonogram, and (C) scintigraphy.

C

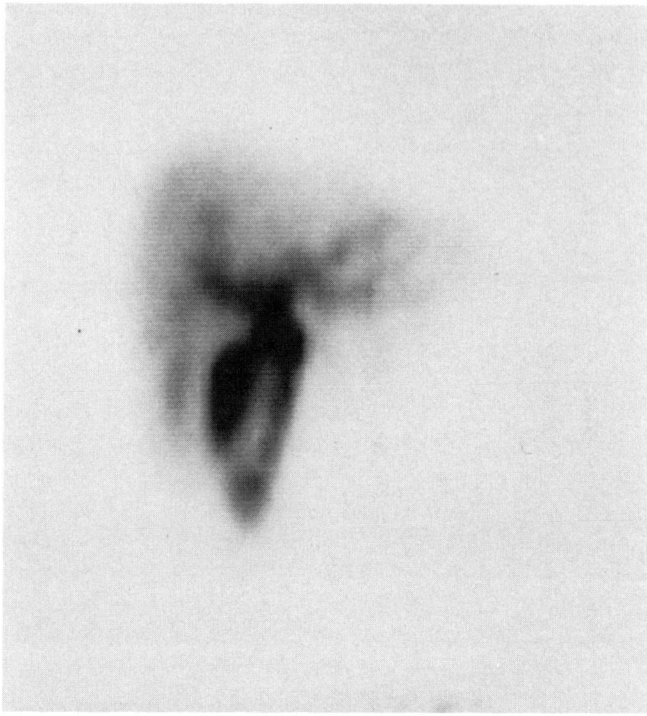

FIGURE 6. *Continued.*

VI. OTHER

A. Suprahepatic[21–27]

The suprahepatic gallbladder is a rare type of gallbladder ectopia, with only a few cases reported (Figure 7). While it may occur in isolation, it is usually associated with hypoplasia of the right hepatic lobe. A suprahepatic gallbladder also has been reported with hepatomegaly due to macronodular cirrhosis.[25] The suprahepatic gallbladder is rarely intrathoracic, associated either with a right diaphragmatic eventration,[24] or a traumatic right diaphragmatic hernia.[27] The suprahepatic gallbladder location may be anterior (Figure 8) or posterior over the dome of the right hepatic lobe. An associated mesentery might explain this unusual suprahepatic location. Reported cases usually have been associated with biliary symptoms. As with the retrohepatic gallbladder, the cystic duct of the suprahepatic gallbladder inserts normally.

There are rare reports of a suprahepatic gallbladder associated with hepatic inversion.[28,29] In one of these cases, the gallbladder was midline, not associated with the falciform ligament. In another, the gallbladder was between the right hepatic lobe and the diaphragm (Figure 9).

B. Wandering, Floating, or Ptotic

The gallbladder normally lies in close apposition to the right hepatic lobe, fixed by the peritoneum. When this peritoneal reflection is incomplete

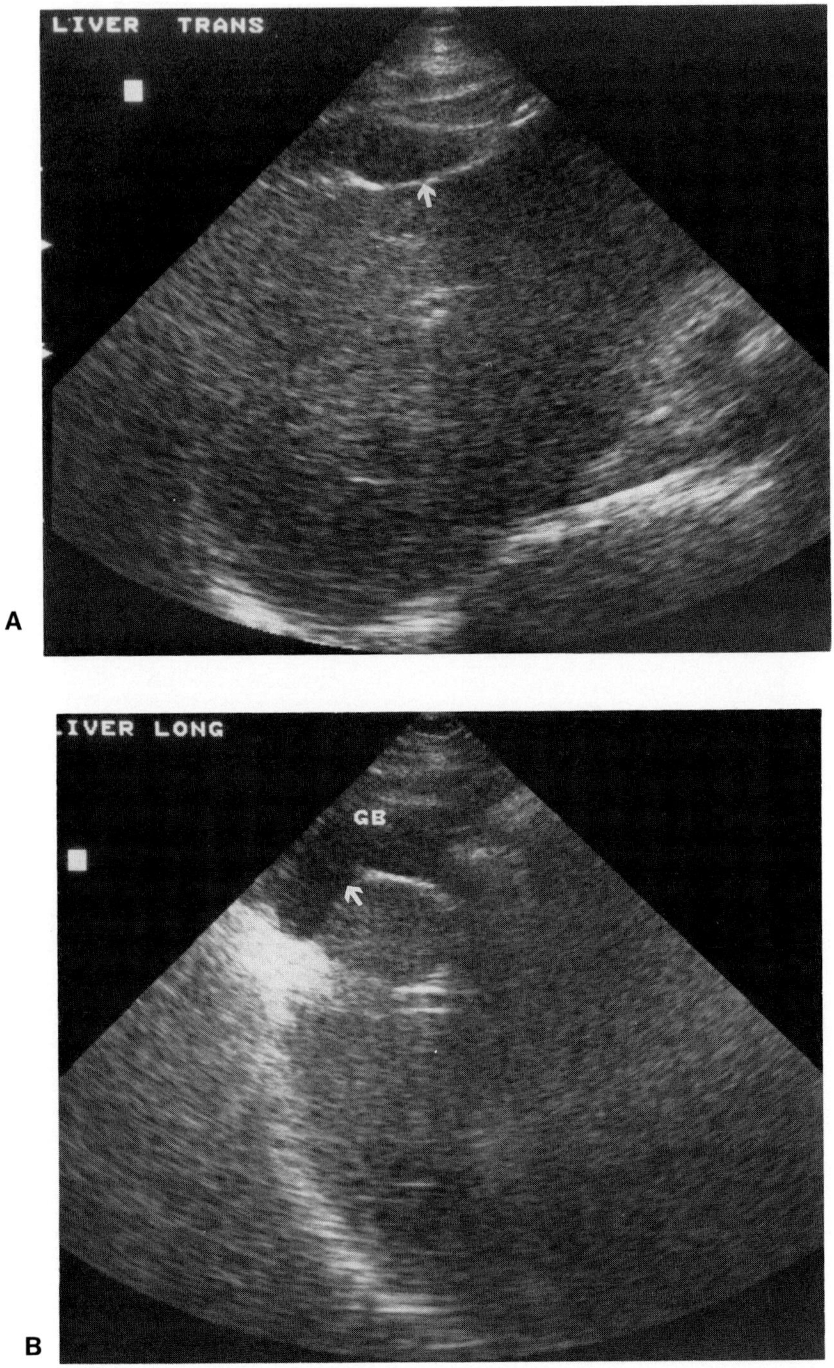

FIGURE 7. Suprahepatic gallbladder (arrow) in a patient with bowel interposed between the liver and the diaphragm (Chilaiditi's syndrome) is shown on (A) transverse and (B) longitudinal sonogram, and (C) and (D) CT images. The bowel causes some artifact on the sonograms.

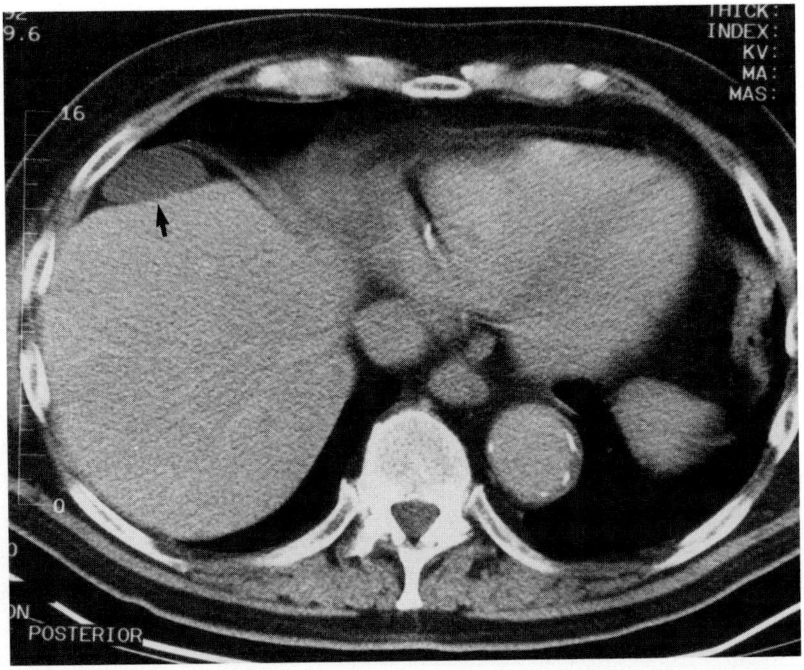

C

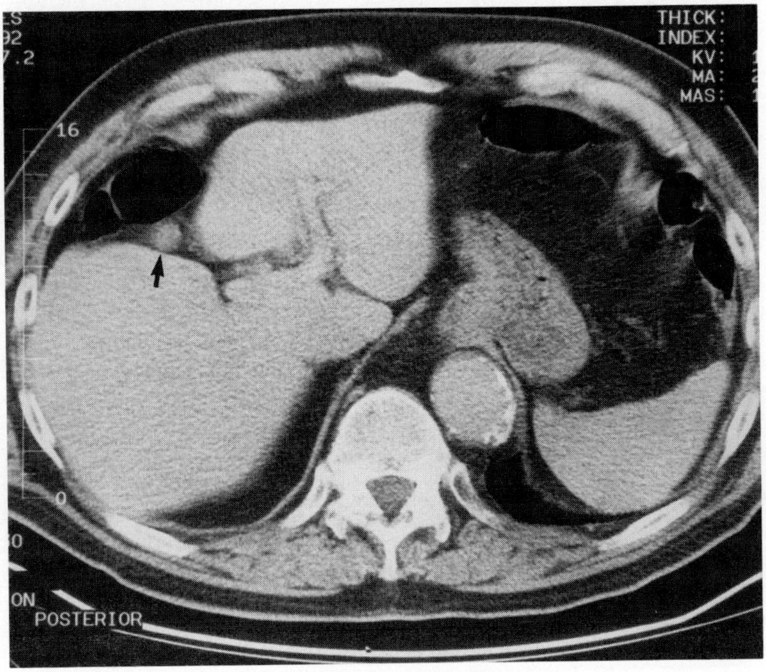

D

FIGURE 7. *Continued.*

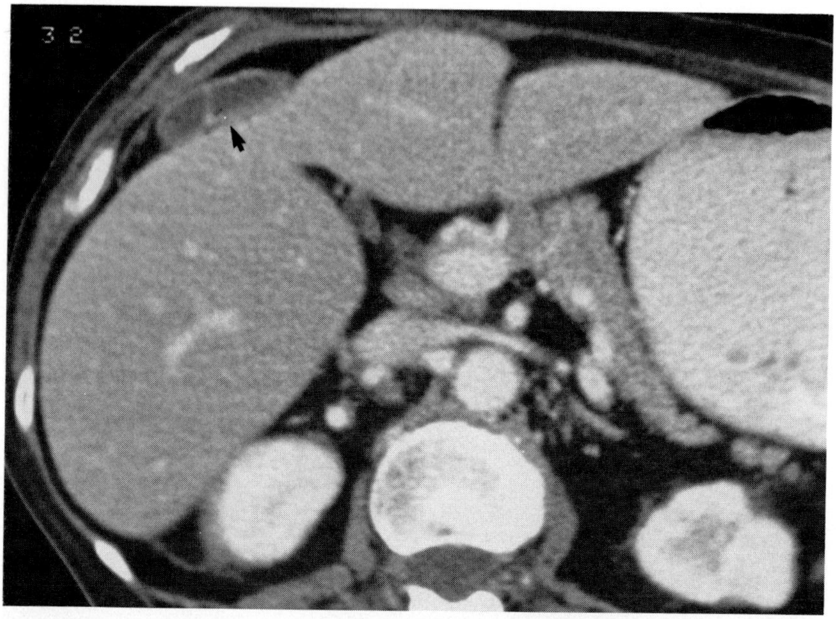

FIGURE 8. CT images of an anterior gallbladder in a 65-year-old female with the gallbladder extending through the interlobar fissure and lying anteriorly to the right hepatic lobe.

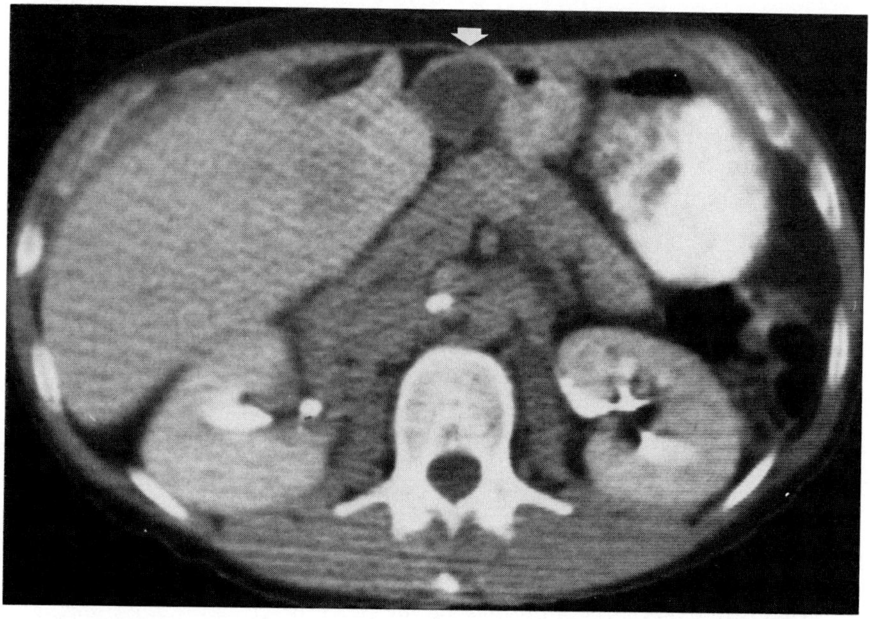

FIGURE 9. Epigastric gallbladder (arrow) is seen in a patient with hepatic inversion. (From Hopper, K. D., *Gastrointest. Radiol.*, 13, 355, 1988. With permission.)

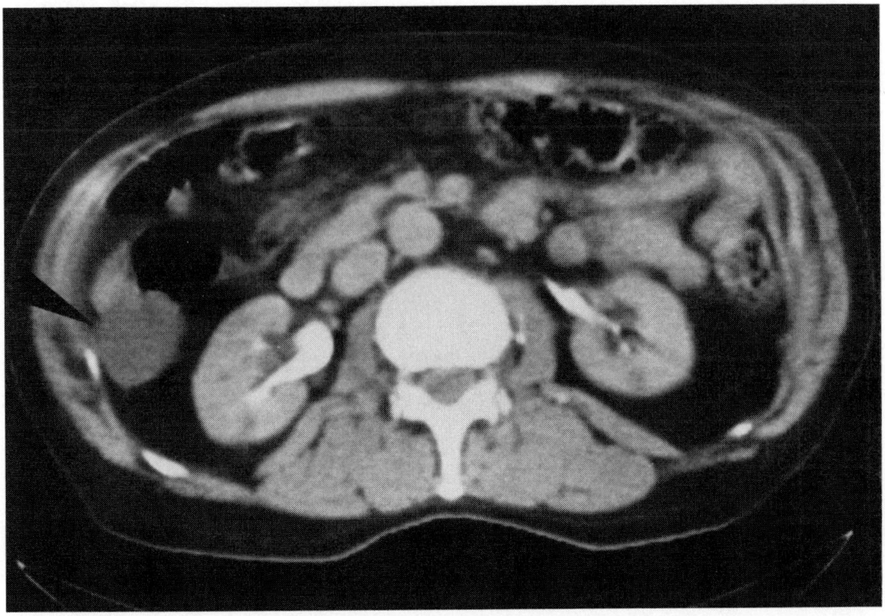

FIGURE 10. CT section through the mid-abdomen demonstrates a ptotic gallbladder (arrowhead) which lies not only caudal to the right hepatic lobe, but lateral and posterior to the ascending colon as well. (From Meilstrup, J. W., Hopper, K. D., and Thieme, G. A., *AJR*, 157, 1205, 1991. With permission.)

or lax, the gallbladder is allowed to "wander" or "float" in the abdomen.[12] This mobility results in many ectopic locations of the gallbladder, including lateral to the liver, adjacent to the pancreas, suprahepatic, retrohepatic, and even pelvic[30,31] (Figures 10 through 14). This variable position of the floating gallbladder can easily mimic disease.

The presence of a mesentery allows the gallbladder to float or hang freely in the peritoneal cavity, sometimes suspended by only a vascular/cystic duct pedicle.[7,32] This variant is present in up to 5% of the population.[33,34] The presence of such a floating gallbladder is important to the surgeon because these patients may develop symptoms in varying abdominal locations, causing a confusing clinical presentation. Additionally, there is the risk of torsion if a mobile, hanging gallbladder twists on its long mesentery.[6,34]

Wandering or floating gallbladders may be seen in several other less common ectopic locations (described below).

1. Epiploic Foramen (of Winslow)

This rare ectopic location may be the rarest of all internal hernias.[35] It has been diagnosed at surgery, but also has been detected on oral cholecystography and upper GI series.[36] A significant number of cases reported in the literature suggest that this ectopic location may not be as rare as originally thought.[37] Symptoms occur typically in the right upper quadrant/

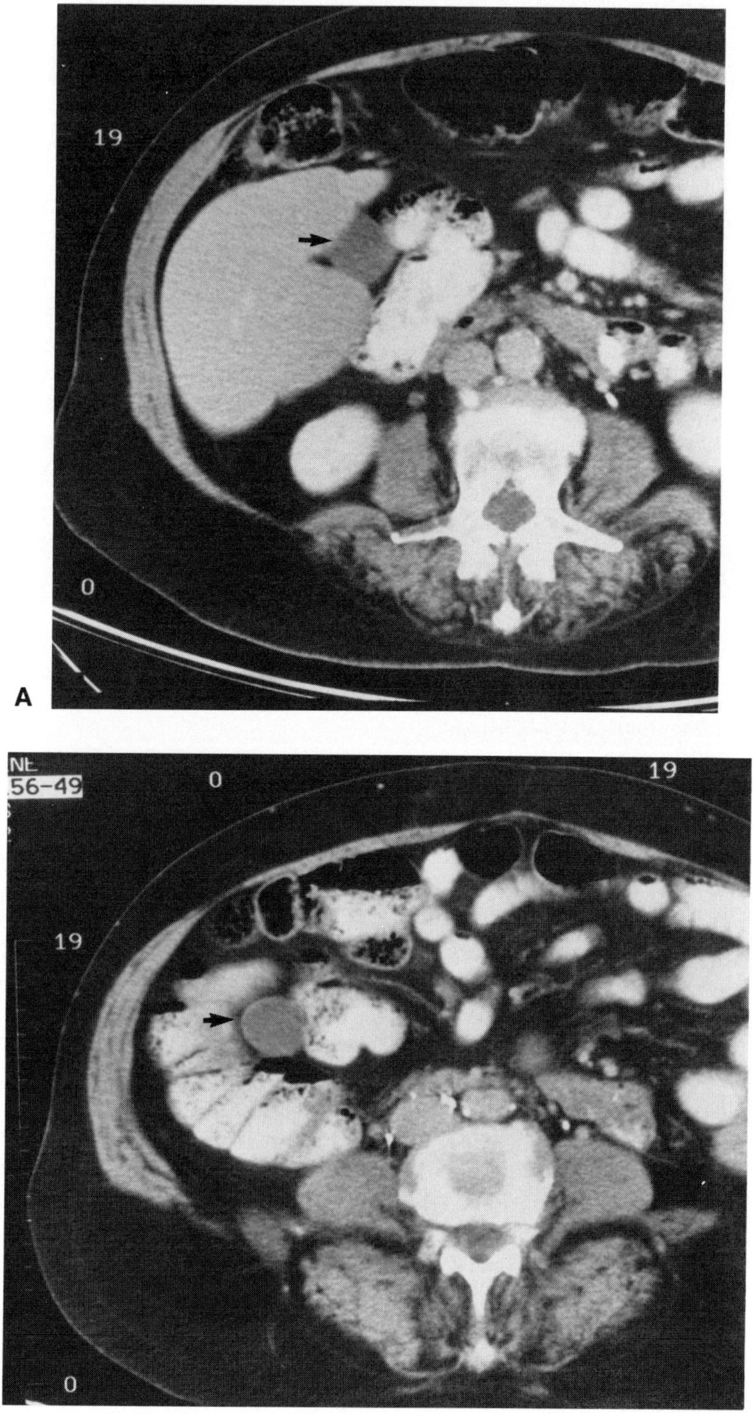

FIGURE 11. (A), (B) ''Hanging'' gallbladder (arrow).

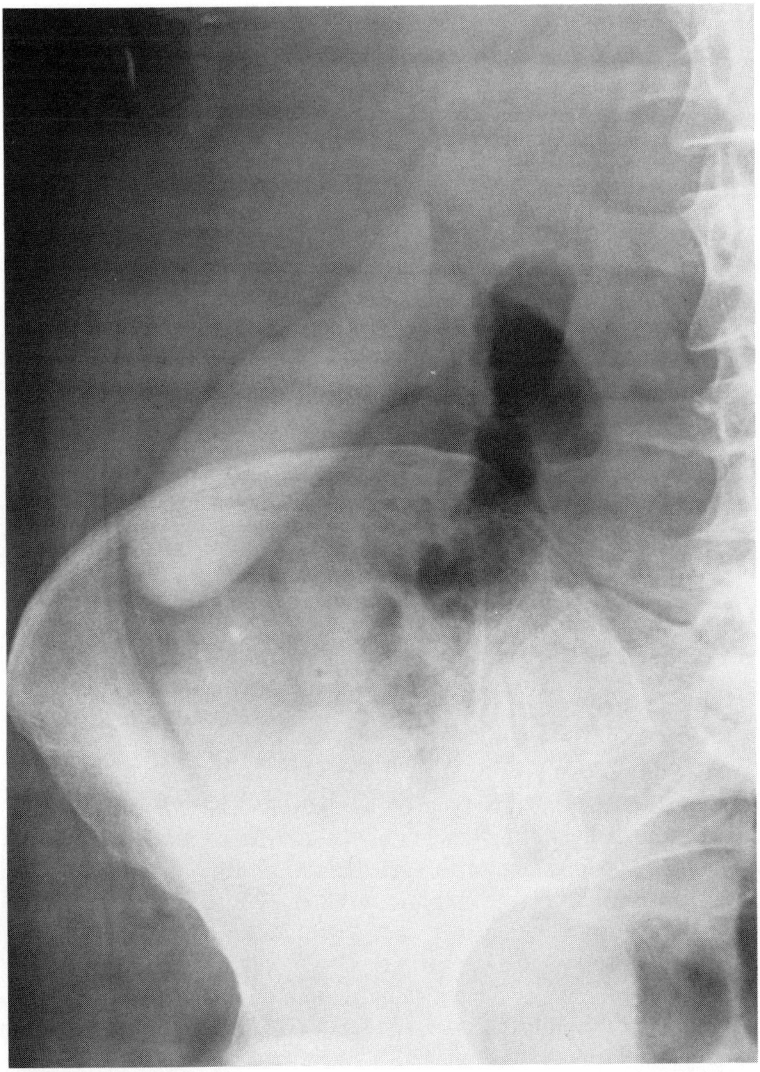

FIGURE 12. Elongated gallbladder in the right pelvis is seen on oral cholecystogram.

mid-epigastric region, and may show some relationship with patient activity and position, such as stooping.[37] On oral cholecystography the gallbladder is displaced, lying medial to the duodenal bulb on frontal views, failing to change position with patient movement or with manual compression.[36] A "draping effect" has been described on oral cholecystography due to the close relationship of the apex of the duodenal bulb and the lesser curvature of the stomach.[37] Almost all cases have been in females. Computed tomography is probably the best modality for diagnosis of this rare hernia because the gallbladder, stomach, and lesser sac relationships are generally well demonstrated.

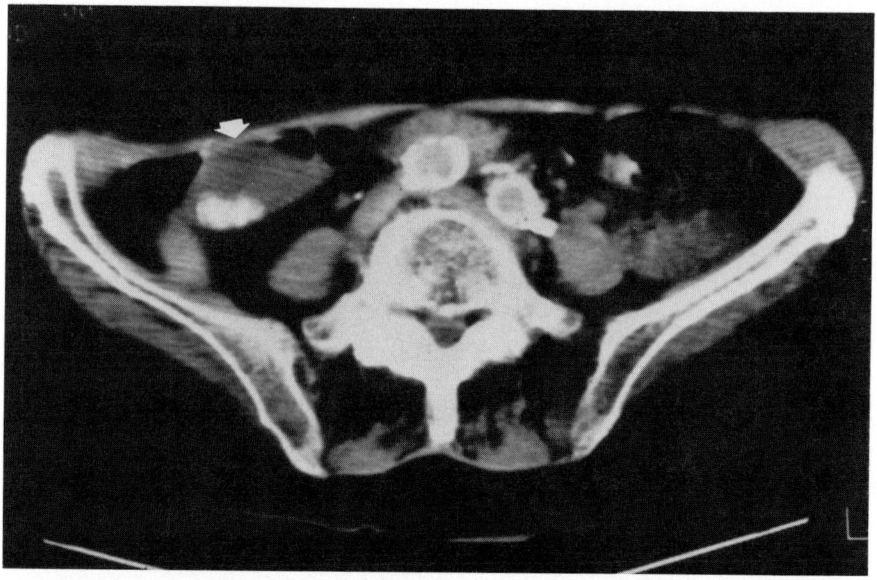

FIGURE 13. Pelvic gallbladder (with gallstones incidentally noted) is demonstrated on this CT image. Sometimes the gallbladder mesentery is long, and the gallbladder can be found far caudad to the right hepatic lobe, and located in the pelvis. (From Meilstrup, J. W., Hopper, K. D., and Thieme, G. A., *AJR*, 157, 1205, 1991. With permission.)

It is postulated that this type of herniation occurs because of a long gallbladder mesentery, which also may be associated with gallbladder volvulus.[38] Predisposing factors to such herniation of a floating gallbladder include an abnormally large epiploic foramen of Winslow and a large right hepatic lobe which positions the gallbladder next to the epiploic foramen.[35,37]

The gallbladder has also been found within the mesocolon; to reach this area, migration through the epiploic foramen and into the omental bursa must have occurred.[39]

2. Retrorenal

The peritoneal cavity can occasionally extend lateral to and even behind the kidney. For this reason, a floating gallbladder can rarely lie lateral and posterior to the kidney, simulating a retroperitoneal or renal lesion.[40]

3. Falciform Ligament

There has been a single report of an ectopic gallbladder lying in the falciform ligament. This case, involving a black male with clinical evidence of an 8-cm mass, was diagnosed at surgery, where a ''cystic pear-shaped structure dangling within the falciform ligament'' was found.[41]

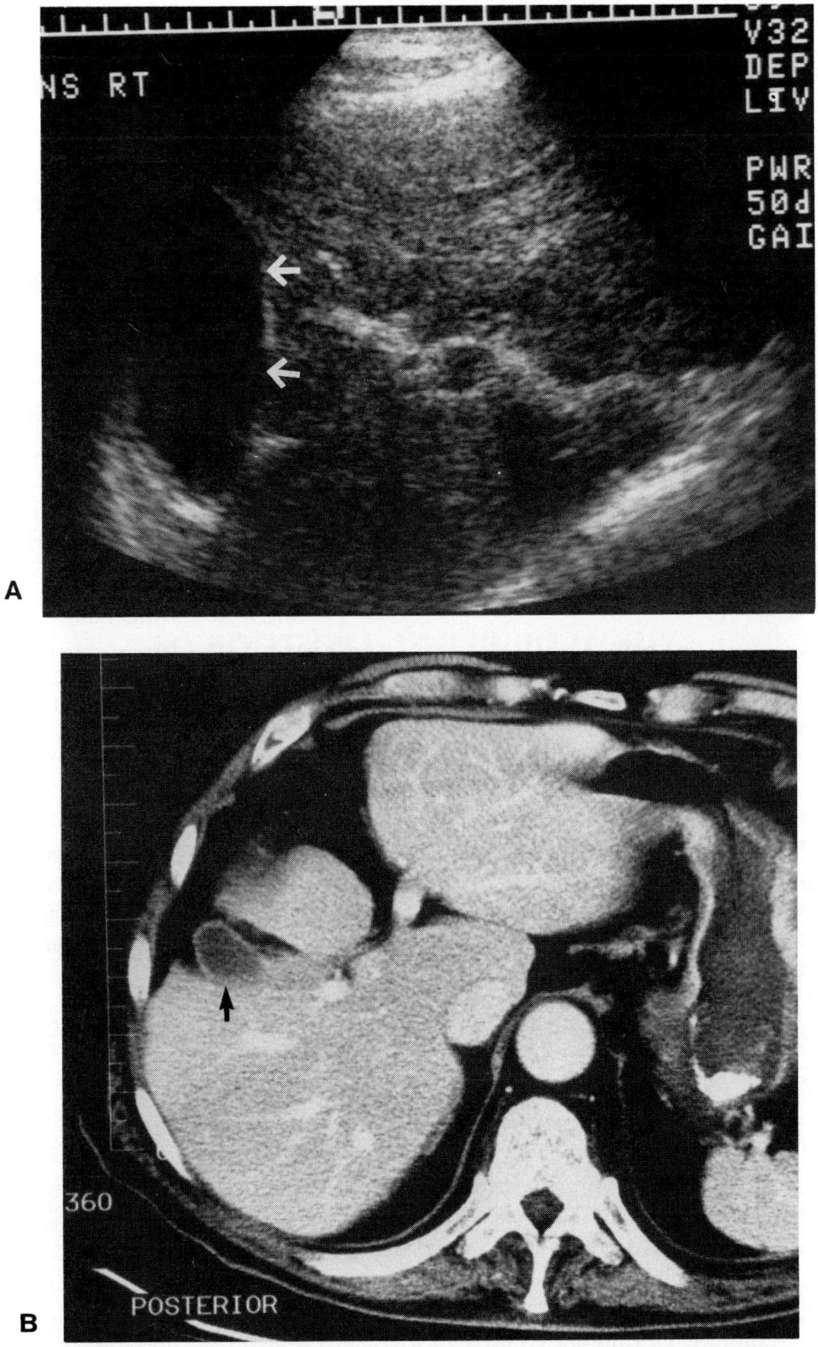

FIGURE 14. Two different examples of the unusual lateral gallbladder (arrows) as demonstrated by sonography on transverse section (A) and CT (B).

4. Extraperitoneal, in Internal Oblique Muscle

At least two cases of the gallbladder lying within the internal oblique muscle of the abdominal wall have been reported. A long mesentery and its loose attachment to the gallbladder were felt to be responsible in one case.[42] The second extraperitoneal gallbladder was described as lying on the internal oblique muscle, splitting the fibers of the external oblique muscle.[43] The patient had presented with a mass below the right ribs which had grown over a period of 2 years.

VII. RELATION TO LIVER ANATOMY

Certain embryologic or developmental changes can cause many of the positional variants of the gallbladder. Agenesis of the right hepatic lobe, for instance, can result in a suprahepatic or retrohepatic gallbladder location; the gallbladder maintains a normal relationship with the medial segment of the left hepatic lobe, which assumes a more posterolateral position because the right lobe is absent.[22,44,45] Separation of the right and left hepatic lobes has been associated with a malpositioned, anterior gallbladder.[46]

VIII. ACQUIRED MALPOSITION OF THE GALLBLADDER

An ectopic position of the gallbladder can be acquired. Because of the close anatomic relationship between the gallbladder and liver, changes in liver positions can affect the gallbladder position. For example, with cirrhosis the interlobar fissure and gallbladder rotate counterclockwise due to atrophy of the right hepatic lobe.[47,48] Other liver changes associated with cirrhosis, such as fatty infiltration, regenerating nodules, or possibly focal fibrosis could result in displacement of the gallbladder from its normal position, mimicking true ectopia.[49]

IX. CONCLUSION

The gallbladder can be located almost anywhere in the abdomen. Whenever the gallbladder is not found in its ''normal'' location, and has not been surgically removed, an ectopic position should be suspected. The diagnosis of an ectopic gallbladder is usually easy with sonography and CT, and its identification can prevent injury from invasive procedures and surgery.[47] Ectopic locations of the gallbladder, therefore, should be carefully documented and communicated to the patient's physician. A knowledge of the more common ectopic locations will also help prevent misdiagnosis when the gallbladder presents as a pseudomass.

REFERENCES

1. **Blanton, D. E., Bream, C. A., and Mandel, S.R.,** Gallbladder ectopia. A review of anomalies of position, *AJR*, 121, 396, 1974.
2. **Velchik, M. G. and Noel, A. W.,** False-positive liver scan due to an intrahepatic gallbladder detected by cholescintigraphy, *Clin. Nucl. Med.*, 12, 50, 1987.
3. **Large, A. M.,** Left-sided gallbladder and liver without situs inversus, *Arch. Surg.*, 87, 120, 1963.
4. **Levin, E. L. and Saksenberg, R.,** Left-sided common bile duct and gallbladder in the absence of situs inversus, *S. Afr. J. Surg.*, 18, 23, 1980.
5. **Duimstra, F. and Greenfield, R. E.,** Left liver lobe gall bladder, *S. D. J. Med.*, 30, 7, 1977.
6. **Haas, G. E., Harris, J. L., and Segal, L. B.,** Situs inversus totalis with calculi in a left-sided gallbladder: report of a case, *J. Am. Osteopath. Assoc.*, 83, 718, 1984.
7. **Corcoran, D. B. and Wallace, K. K.,** Congenital anomalies of the gallbladder, *Am. Surg.*, 20, 709, 1954.
8. **Bleich, A. R., Hamblin, D. O., and Martin, D.,** Left-upper-quadrant gallbladder, *JAMA*, 147, 849, 1951.
9. **Etter, L. E.,** Left-sided gallbladder. Necessity for film of the entire abdomen in cholecystography, *Am. J. Roentgenol.*, 70, 987, 1953.
10. **Herrington, J. L.,** Gallbladder arising from the left hepatic lobe, *Am. J. Surg.*, 112, 106, 1966.
11. **Korn, O., Csendes, A., and Bastias, J.,** Anomalies of extrahepatic biliary duct and gallbladder associated with intestinal malrotation: a case report, *Surgery*, 103, 496, 1988.
12. **Hatfield, P. M. and Wise, R. E.,** Anatomic variation in the gallbladder and bile ducts, *Semin. Roentgenol.*, 11, 157, 1976.
13. **Schachner, A.,** Anomalies of the gall-bladder and bile-passages, *Ann. Surg.*, 64, 419, 1916.
14. **Banzo, I., Carril, J. M., Arnal, C., and Quirce, R.,** Left-sided gallbladder. An incidental finding on hepatobiliary scintigraphy, *Clin. Nucl. Med.*, 15, 358, 1990.
15. **McNamee, E. P.,** Intrahepatic gallbladder, *AJR*, 33, 603, 1935.
16. **Gross, R. E.,** Congenital anomalies of the gallbladder, *Arch. Surg.*, 32, 131, 1936.
17. **Schneider, E. A., Eisner, M., and Fridrich, R.,** Scintigraphic demonstration of an intrahepatic gall-bladder presenting as a focal liver lesion, *Br. J. Radiol.*, 52, 754, 1979.
18. **Dumont, M. and Danais, S.,** Intrahepatic gallbladder simulating choledochal cyst on DISIDA scintigraphy, *Clin. Nucl. Med.*, 9, 657, 1984.
19. **Lloyd, T. V.,** Empyema of an intrahepatic gallbladder, *Clin. Nucl. Med.*, 4, 341, 1979.
20. **Greaves, F. W., Nguyen, K. T., and Sauerbrei, E. E.,** Retrohepatic gallbladder diagnosed by sonography and scintigraphy, *J. Can. Assoc. Radiol.*, 34, 319, 1983.
21. **Youngwirth, L. D., Peters, J. C., and Perry, M. C.,** The suprahepatic gallbladder, *Radiology*, 149, 57, 1983.
22. **Faintuch, J., Machado, M. C. C., and Raia, A. A.,** Suprahepatic gallbladder with hypoplasia of the right lobe of the liver, *Arch. Surg.*, 115, 658, 1980.
23. **Allison, M. C., Milkins, S., Burroughs, A. K., Rogers, H. S., and Thomas, H. C.,** Bronchobiliary fistula due to acute cholecystitis in a suprahepatic gall bladder, *Postgrad. Med. J.*, 63, 291, 1987.
24. **Anderson, R. D., Connell, T. H., and Lowman, R. M.,** Inversion of the liver and suprahepatic gallbladder associated with eventration of the diaphragm, *Radiology*, 97, 87, 1970.
25. **Van Gansbeke, D., de Toeuf, J., Cremer, M., Engelholm, L., and Struyven, J.,** Suprahepatic gallbladder: a rare congenital anomaly, *Gastrointest. Radiol.*, 9, 341, 1984.

26. **Organ, C. H. and Hayes, D. F.,** Supradiaphragmatic right liver lobe and gallbladder, *Arch. Surg.*, 115, 989, 1980.
27. **Keene, C. H. and Copleman, B.,** Traumatic right diaphragmatic hernia. Case with delayed herniation of the liver and gallbladder, *Ann. Surg.*, 122, 191, 1945.
28. **Hopper, K. D.,** Hepatic inversion with an epigastric gallbladder, *Gastrointest. Radiol.*, 13, 355, 1988.
29. **Leekam, R. N., Ilves, R., and Shankar, L.,** Inversion of gallbladder secondary to traumatic herniation of liver: CT findings, *J. Comput. Assist. Tomogr.*, 11, 163, 1987.
30. **Morse, J. M. D., Lakshman, S., and Thomas, E.,** Gallbladder ectopia simulating pancreatic mass on CT, *Gastrointest. Radiol.*, 10, 111, 1985.
31. **Pradeep, V. M., Ramachandran, K., and Sasidharan, K.,** Anomalous position of the gallbladder: ultrasonographic and scintigraphic demonstration in four cases, *J. Clin. Ultrasound*, 20, 593, 1992.
32. **Regen, J. F. and Poindexter, A.,** Suprahepatic position of the gallbladder, *Arch. Surg.*, 90, 175, 1965.
33. **Gross, R. E.,** Congenital anomalies of the gallbladder. A review of one hundred and forty-eight cases, with report of a double gallbladder, *Arch. Surg.*, 32, 131, 1936.
34. **Merine, D., Meziane, M., and Fishman, E. K.,** CT diagnosis of gallbladder torsion, *J. Comput. Assist. Tomogr.*, 11, 712, 1987.
35. **Borkar, B. B., Whelan, J. G., and Creech, J. L.,** Herniation of the gallbladder through the foramen of Winslow, *Dig. Dis. Sci.*, 25, 228, 1980.
36. **Vint, W. A.,** Herniation of the gallbladder through the epiploic foramen into the lesser sac: radiologic diagnosis, *Radiology*, 86, 1035, 1966.
37. **Dardik, H. and Cowen, R.,** Herniation of the gallbladder through the epiploic foramen into the lesser sac, *Ann. Surg.*, 165, 644, 1967.
38. **Bach, D. B., Satin, R., Palayew, M., Lisbona, R., and Tessler, F.,** Herniation and strangulation of the gallbladder through the foramen of Winslow, *AJR*, 142, 541, 1984.
39. **Bilton, J. L. and Huggins, C. L.,** Anomaly of the gallbladder, *Ohio St. Med. J.*, 62, 1034, 1966.
40. **Ehman, R. L. and Morrish, H. F.,** Retrorenal gallbladder. A case report, *J. Can. Assoc. Radiol.*, 34, 321, 1983.
41. **Nelson, P. A., Schmitz, R. A., and Perutsea, S.,** Anomalous position of the gall bladder within the falciform ligament, *AMA Arch. Surg.*, 66, 679, 1953.
42. **Alawaneh, I.,** Anomaly of the gallbladder lying extraperitoneally in the internal oblique muscle: report of an unusual case, *Int. Surg.*, 64, 45, 1979.
43. **Bullard, R. W.,** Subcutaneous or extraperitoneal gallbladder, *JAMA*, 129, 949, 1945.
44. **Radin, D. R., Colletti, P. M., Ralls, P. W., Boswell, W. D., and Halls, J. M.,** Agenesis of the right lobe of the liver, *Radiology*, 164, 639, 1987.
45. **Radin, D. R.,** Letter to the editor, *Gastrointest. Radiol.*, 14, 363, 1989.
46. **Taqi, S.,** Congenital anomaly of the liver and gall bladder, *J. Pakistan Med. Assoc.*, August, 202, 1987.
47. **Gore, R. M., Ghahremani, G. G., Joseph, A. E., Nemcek, A. A., Jr., Marn, C. S., and Vogelzang, R. L.,** Acquired malposition of the colon and gallbladder in patients with cirrhosis: CT findings and clinical implications, *Radiology*, 171, 739, 1989.
48. **Nardi, P. M., Yaghoobian, J., and Ruchman, R. B.,** CT demonstration of retrohepatic gallbladder in severe cirrhosis, *J. Comput. Assist. Tomogr.*, 12, 968, 1988.
49. **Owshalimpur, D. and Karimeddini, M. K.,** Gallbladder displacement in a cirrhotic patient simulating ectopia, *Clin. Nucl. Med.*, 6, 284, 1982.

Chapter 6

VARIATIONS OF NUMBER

Claudia J. Kasales and Jon W. Meilstrup

TABLE OF CONTENTS

0–8493–4788–2/94/$0.00+$.50

I. INTRODUCTION

Congenital anomalies of the gallbladder are rare; however, knowledge of such malformations is extremely important in the practice of both radiology and surgery.[1] In 1926, prompted by the development of new methods for visualizing the gallbladder (such as oral cholecystography), Boyden[2] published an extensive review of mammalian gallbladder anomalies. Ten years later Gross[3] reviewed 148 cases of congenital anomalies of the gallbladder, concentrating on variants noted in humans. Their work remains the backbone for the classification of gallbladder anomalies, and forms the basis of the following discussion.

II. GALLBLADDER DUPLICATION

Duplication of the gallbladder is relatively rare in humans, with a reported incidence of 1:3000 to 4000.[2] The radiologic manifestations were first described in 1926 by Nichols,[4] who noted two distinct rows of calculi in the region of the gallbladder on the abdominal radiograph of a patient complaining of intermittent right upper quadrant pain. At surgery a duplicated gallbladder was noted, with stones in each sac. In the late 1920s and early 1930s the popularization of methods to visualize the gallbladder prompted the discovery of several additional cases of gallbladder duplication, however, the radiologic and operative descriptions of the anomalies were often insufficient to allow accurate categorization. More recently, duplicated gallbladders have been diagnosed with scintigraphy,[5] T-tube cholangiography,[6] endoscopic retrograde cholangiography,[7,8] and sonography.[9,10]

The spectrum of gallbladder duplication is broad. Incomplete longitudinal division of the gallbladder results in the bilobed or partially divided gallbladder. True duplication, however, is usually present in one of two forms: the true double gallbladder and the H-shaped (or accessory) gallbladder.

Two main types of bilobed or partially subdivided gallbladder have been described. In the first, the gallbladder has a normal external appearance, but is divided into two communicating cavities by a longitudinal fibrous septum that may contain muscular or glandular elements (Figure 1A). In the second type, the division of the gallbladder is evident upon external inspection. The gallbladder appears V-shaped, with both cavities separated toward the fundus and fused at the base (Figure 1B). In both types of duplication a single cystic duct is present, which distinguishes this anomaly from the true double gallbladder and the H-shaped gallbladder. The bilobed gallbladder is thought to result from the longitudinal splitting or incomplete vacuolation of the organ during its solid stage of embryogenesis. It is

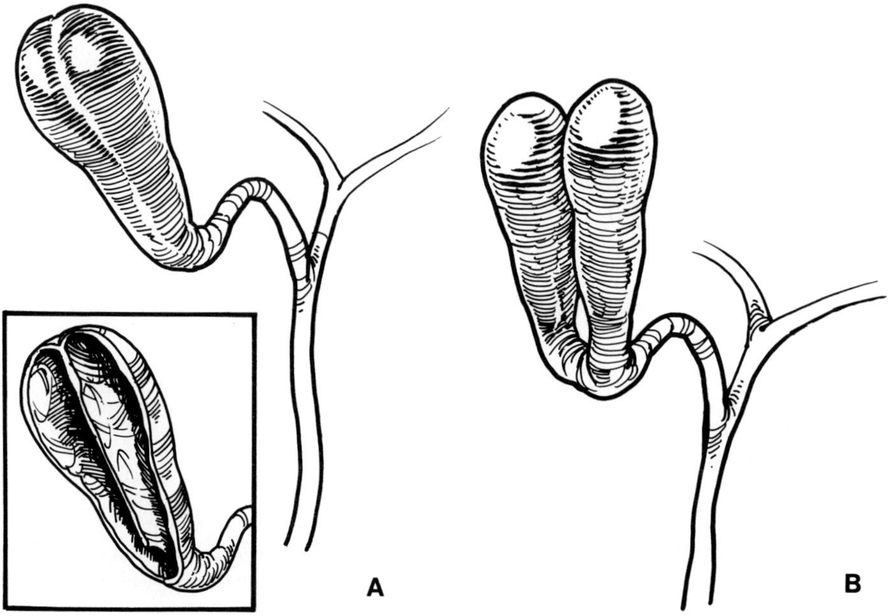

FIGURE 1. (A) One form of bilobed gallbladder has a normal external appearance. The communicating cavities are separated by a longitudinal fibrous septum, evident upon dissection (inset). (B) The second form of bilobed gallbladder appears V-shaped, with both cavities fused at the base, drained by a single cystic duct. (Modified from Ross, R. J. and Sachs, M. D., *Am. J. Roentgenol.*, 104, 656, 1968. With permission.)

difficult to diagnose radiographically because it requires the visualization of a single cystic duct emanating from the duplicated viscus.

The true double or Y-shaped gallbladder (Figure 2A) consists of two individual gallbladders with separate cystic ducts that join prior to entering the biliary system.[2] The H-shaped gallbladder, on the other hand, is structurally different (Figure 2B), consisting of an organ of normal size, shape, and position (located within the gallbladder fossa) accompanied by another ''accessory'' gallbladder whose cystic duct empties separately into the biliary tree. In both forms of duplication the accessory vesicle is usually the same size or smaller than the normal gallbladder and, in the H-shaped variant, can be located outside of the gallbladder fossa. Unlike the bilobed gallbladder, the Y- and H-shaped gallbladder result from the persistence of duct buds that develop either along the cystic duct (resulting in the Y-shaped gallbladder) or from another section of the biliary system (resulting in the H-shaped gallbladder).[3]

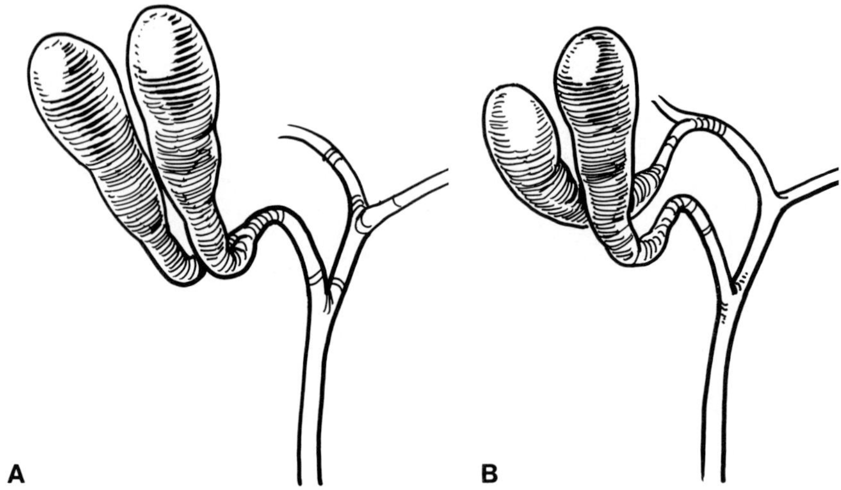

FIGURE 2. True duplication of the gallbladder presents as one of two forms. (A) The Y-shaped gallbladder consists of two gallbladders with separate cystic ducts that fuse prior to joining the common bile duct. (B) The H-shaped gallbladder consists of two organs with individual cystic ducts draining separately into the biliary system. (Modified from Ross, R. J. and Sachs, M. D., *Am. J. Roentgenol.*, 104, 656, 1968. With permission.)

Stone disease is a common finding in duplicated gallbladders, and is often what brings the anomaly to the attention of a physician. In a review of 207 reports of gallbladder duplication,[10] calculi were present in 50% of bilobed duplications, 79% of Y-shaped duplications, and 95% of H-shaped duplications. In 26 of 90 cases only one of the sacs was involved. Accompanying inflammatory changes (including cholecystitis and empyema) have also been reported,[11,12] as well as involvement with adenocarcinoma, adenomyosis, and torsion. Whether duplicated gallbladders have an increased prevalence of disease, however, is debated.[3,11,13]

The significance of the duplicated gallbladder is evident in the patient with abdominal pain or symptoms of biliary tract disease. Radiologic examinations that assess patency of the cystic duct [such as oral cholecystography, endoscopic retrograde cholecystopancreatography (ERCP), T-tube cholangiography, or scintigraphy] can detect gallbladder duplication.[5–8,14] Such studies in a symptomatic patient, however, may be falsely negative if a second gallbladder with an open cystic duct is present.[12] Similarly, a patient with unrecognized gallbladder duplication who has undergone previous cholecystectomy may present with recurrent symptoms of

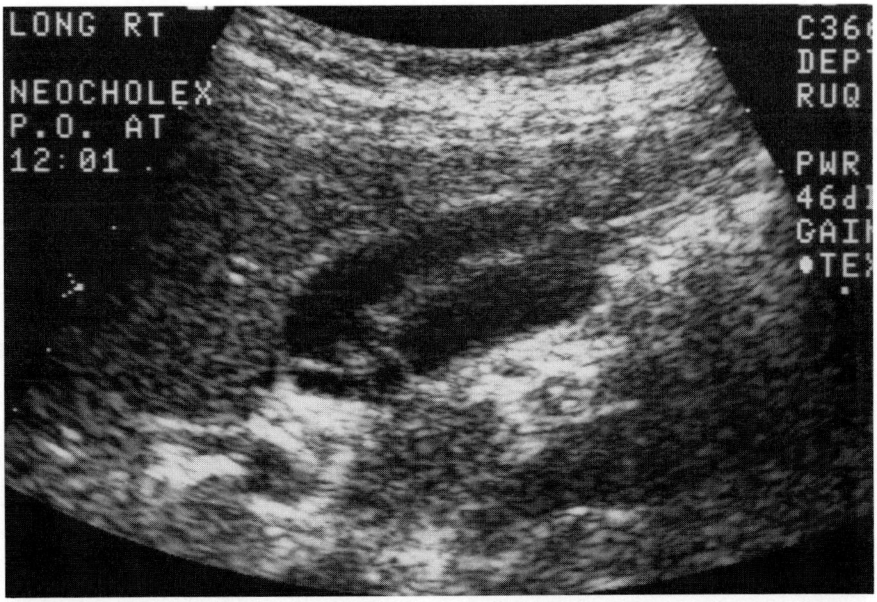

A

FIGURE 3. Sonography of duplicated gallbladder, proven by laparoscopic surgery. Longitudinal (A) and transverse (B) views. No significant change in the gallbladder appearance was noted after administering a fatty meal.

cholecystitis due to involvement of the second viscus. Unless the second gallbladder is visualized, the patient's symptoms may be falsely attributed to other causes such as post-cholecystectomy syndrome. Cross-sectional imaging studies [sonography and computed tomography, (CT)] may more readily assess the presence of a second viscus[16] (Figure 3).

Several mimics of gallbladder duplication have been described in the literature. One of the most common is the tightly curved, tortuous gallbladder. This atypical shape can cause the gallbladder to appear as two lumens on transverse ultrasound imaging; longitudinal views, however, demonstrate the presence of a single viscus.[17] Gallbladder septations might also resemble gallbladder duplication on some views.[18] Occasionally Ladd's bands can traverse the gallbladder, causing a deep ridge that also mimics a duplicated gallbladder.[18] Duplication of the duodenum rarely has been confused with a duplicated gallbladder.[19]

Gallbladder duplication can also be misinterpreted as other entities. On oral cholecystography a second viscus can be misinterpreted as overlapping

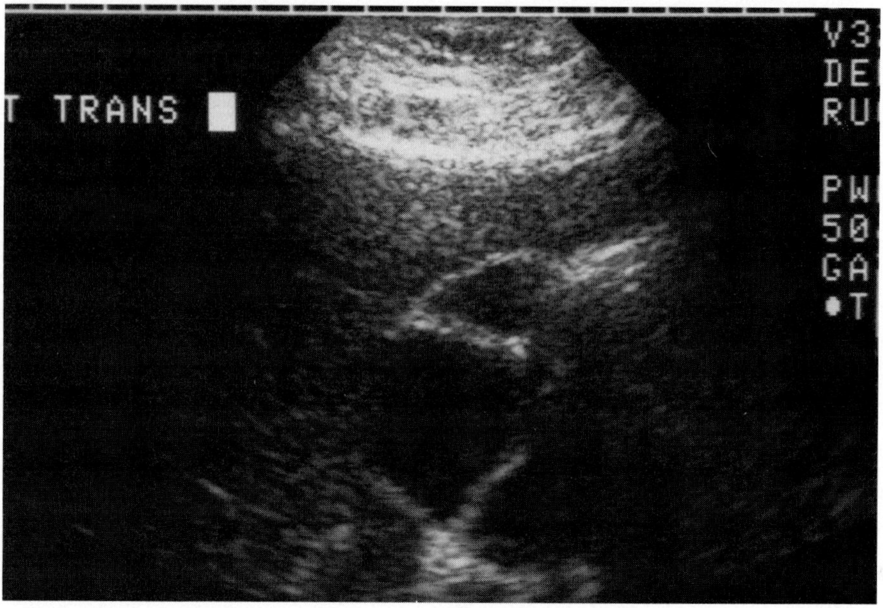

B

FIGURE 3. *Continued.*

portions of a tortuous gallbladder.[4,9] A duplicated gallbladder can also be mistaken for a septated or folded gallbladder.[17,18] By remaining aware of the many variations in the appearance of the gallbladder, such misdiagnosis can be avoided.

III. GALLBLADDER TRIPLICATION

Gallbladder triplication is extremely rare in humans. Generally three main types have been described, which vary according to the number of cystic ducts and their insertion.[20] One type has three vesicles and three cystic ducts that fuse to form a common cystic duct before joining the common bile duct (Figure 4A). In the second type the cystic duct of two gallbladders fuse before joining the common duct, while the cystic duct of the third gallbladder enters the common duct separately (Figure 4B). The third type consists of three vesicles whose individual cystic ducts join the common duct at separate locations (Figure 4C).

Embryologically the triple gallbladder is felt to result from the persistence of multiple duct buds. As in gallbladder duplication, a higher incidence of pathology may occur in gallbladder triplication.[21] Although rare, radiographic findings of gallbladder triplication have been reported.[22]

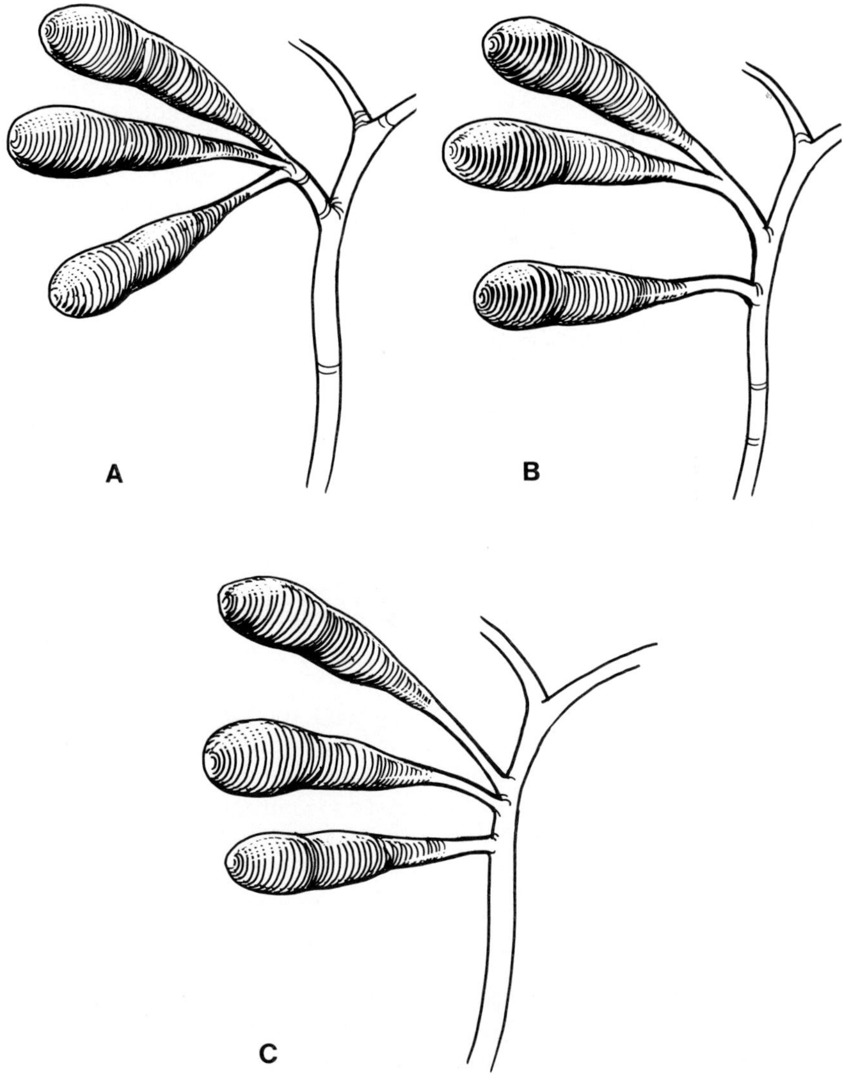

FIGURE 4. Three main types of gallbladder triplication have been described. In the first (A), three cystic ducts fuse to form a common cystic duct prior to joining the common bile duct. In the second form (B), two cystic ducts fuse before joining the common bile duct while the third drains separately. In the third form (C), the cystic duct of each vesicle drains into the common bile duct separately. (Modified from Ross, R. J. and Sachs, M. D., *Am. J. Roentgenol.*, 104, 656, 1968. With permission.)

IV. AGENESIS OF THE GALLBLADDER

Complete agenesis of the gallbladder is extremely rare, occurring in <1 in 6000 live births.[23–25] Although the exact cause is not known, this anomaly is thought to result either from failure of the cystic bud to form, or from lack of vacuolation. A strong female predominance is present in cases discovered at surgery, however, autopsy surveys generally show an equal prevalence in males and females.[25]

There appear to be two broad populations of patients with gallbladder agenesis.[23] In the first group, usually discovered during childhood, additional anomalies are present coincident with gallbladder agenesis.[23] In one autopsy series of 181 cases of gallbladder agenesis, 65% were associated with one or more congenital anomalies.[25] A retrospective autopsy study[26] further divided this group with anomalies into those with multiple other anomalies involving the genitourinary tract, skeletal system, cardiovascular system, and gastrointestinal tract, and a second smaller subgroup accompanied by only cardiac anomalies or anterior abdominal wall defects. In these patients the associated anomalies are often severe, resulting in early death.

The second broad population consists of those discovered at surgery. These patients tend to have no other congenital anomalies and remain asymptomatic until adulthood when up to 58% have been reported to develop vague symptoms suggestive of biliary tract disease[27] including nausea, vomiting, abdominal bloating, and fatty food intolerance.[28] Up to 50% of these patients have common bile duct stones, and the common duct rarely can be dilated at surgery.[29] Increased tone of the sphincter of Oddi has been proposed as a possible mechanism leading to dilatation of the duct and subsequent stone formation due to stasis, similar to that noted in post-cholecystectomy patients.[22,27,30] Abdominal symptoms in these patients may result from the presence of calculi within the duct or from biliary dyskinesis.[27]

The role of radiology in the diagnosis of gallbladder agenesis is unclear. Congenital absence of the gallbladder has been described as a cause of false positive hepatobiliary sonography and scintigraphy.[31–33] Nonvisualization of the gallbladder in these patients is frequently attributed to gallbladder disease at initial presentation. At surgery, however, the gallbladder cannot be located in its usual position. Intraoperative cholangiography and/or thorough dissection of the extrahepatic ducts may be required to exclude an ectopic location of the organ, and to accurately diagnose gallbladder agenesis.[34,35] Imaging modalities such as ultrasound and CT may suggest the diagnosis,[36,37] however, other causes of a nonvisualized gallbladder would need to be excluded, such as atrophy due to adhesions or gallbladder inflammation and prior cholecystectomy.[28]

Agenesis of the gallbladder has been described in association with other anomalies after *in utero* exposure to thalidomide.[38] In addition, several cases have been published in which multiple family members were affected, suggesting a hereditary trait.[39–42] However, in the majority of cases, it is a sporadic anomaly.[26]

REFERENCES

1 **Schachner, A.,** Anomalies of the gall-bladder and bile-passages, *Ann. Surg.*, 64, 419, 1916.
2. **Boyden, E. A.,** The accessory gall-bladder—an embryological and comparative study of aberrant biliary vesicles occurring in man and the domestic mammals, *Am. J. Anat.*, 38(2), 177, 1926.
3. **Gross, R. E.,** Congenital anomalies of the gallbladder, *Arch. Surg.*, 32, 131, 1936.
4. **Nichols, B. H.,** Double gallbladder, *Radiology*, 6, 255, 1926.
5. **Singh, A., Holmes, R. A., and Witten, D. M.,** Scintigraphic demonstration of a gallbladder anomaly, *AJR*, 144, 77, 1985.
6. **Milner, S. M. and Hawthorn, I. E.,** Double gallbladder diagnosed by T-tube cholangiogram, *J. R. Army Med. Corps*, 135, 84, 1989.
7. **Urbain, D., Jeanmart, J., Janne, P., Lemone, M., Platteborse, R., De Reuck, M., and Delteune, M.,** Double gallbladder with transient cholestasis: preoperative demonstration by endoscopic retrograde cholangiopancreatography, *Gastrointest. Endosc.*, 35, 346, 1989.
8. **Janson, J. A., Gulliver, D., and Cotton, P. B.,** Choledocholithiasis and a double gallbladder, *Gastrointest. Endosc.*, 38, 377, 1992.
9. **Garfield, H. D., Lyons, E. A., and Clifford, S. L.,** Sonographic findings in double gallbladder with cholelithiasis of both lobes, *J. Ultrasound Med.*, 7, 589, 1988.
10. **Peters, M. J. and Cooperberg, P. L.,** Sonography of gallbladder duplication and differential considerations, *AJR*, 145, 241, 1985.
11. **Harlaftis, N., Gray, S. W., and Skandalakis, J. E.,** Multiple gallbladders, *Surg., Gynecol., Obstet.*, 145, 928, 1977.
12. **Cunningham, J. J.,** Empyema of a duplicated gallbladder: echographic findings, *J. Clin. Ultrasound*, 8, 511, 1980.
13. **Guyer, P. B. and McLaughlin, M.,** Congenital double gall-bladder, *Br. J. Radiol.*, 40, 214, 1967.
14. **McDonald, K. and Lwin, T.,** Sonographic and scintigraphic evaluation of gallbladder duplication, *Clin. Nucl. Med.*, 11, 692, 1986.
15. Reference deleted in proof.
16. **Tobias, M. E.,** Letter to the editor. Duplicated gall bladder and situs inversus: findings on sonography and scintigraphy, *AJR*, 159, 1346, 1992.
17. **Goiney, R. C., Schoenecker, S. A., Cyr, D. R., Shuman, W. P., Peters, M. J., and Cooperberg, P. L.,** Sonography of gallbladder duplication and differential considerations, *AJR*, 145, 241, 1985.
18. **Schubert, F. and Jeavons, S.,** Double gallbladder, *Aust. Radiol.*, 29, 343, 1985.
19. **Wrenn, E. L. and Favara, B. E.,** Duodenal duplication (or pancreatic bladder) presenting as double gallbladder, *Surgery*, 69, 858, 1971.

20. **Foster, D. R.,** Triple gallbladder, *Br. J. Radiol.*, 54, 817, 1981.
21. **Kurzweg, F. T. and Cole, P. A.,** Triplication of the gallbladder: review of literature and report of a case, *Am. Surg.*, 45, 410, 1979.
22. **Ross, R. J. and Sachs, M. D.,** Triplication of the gallbladder, *Am. J. Roentgenol.*, 104, 656, 1968.
23. **Jackson, R. J. and McClellan, D.,** Agenesis of the gallbladder. A cause of false-positive ultrasonography, *Am. Surg.*, 55, 36, 1989.
24. **Turkel, S. B., Swanson, V., and Chandrasoma, P.,** Malformations associated with congenital absence of the gall bladder, *J. Med. Gen.*, 20, 445, 1983.
25. **Monroe, S. E.,** Congenital absence of the gallbladder: a statistical study, *J. Int. Coll. Surg.*, 32, 369, 1959.
26. **Beckroittuckel, S., Swanson, V., and Chanohasoma, P.,** Malformations associated with congenital absence of the gallbladder, *J. Med. Gen.*, 20, 445, 1983.
27. **Dixon, C. F. and Lichtman, A. L.,** Congenital absence of the gallbladder, *Surgery*, 17, 11, 1945.
28. **Sanders, G. D., Flores, T., and Arriola, P.,** Congenital absence of the gallbladder and cystic duct: a review of the literature and report of a case, *Am. Surg.*, 54(10), 750, 1968.
29. **Brezing, H. J. and Sanchez, S. M.,** Congenital absence of gallbladder, *N. Y. State J. Med.*, 64, 914, 1964.
30. **Toouli, J., Roberts-Thomson, C., Dent, J., and Lee, J.,** Manometric disorders in patients with suspected sphincter of Oddi dysfunction, *Gastroenterology*, 88, 1243, 1985.
31. **Warshauer, D. M. and Sulzer, J. L.,** Agenesis of the gallbladder. A rare cause for a false-positive hepatobiliary image, *Clin. Nucl. Med.*, 13, 468, 1988.
32. **Dickinson, C. Z., Powers, T. A., Sandler, M. P., and Partain, C. L.,** Congenital absence of the gallbladder: another cause of false-positive hepatobiliary image, *J. Nucl. Med.* 25, 70, 1984.
33. **Jackson, R. J. and McClellan, D.,** Agenesis of the gallbladder. A cause of false positive ultrasonography, *Am. Surg.*, 55, 36, 1989.
34. **Frey, C., Bizer, L., and Ernst, C.,** Agenesis of the gallbladder, *Am. J. Surg.*, 114, 917, 1967.
35. **Kennard, G. K.,** Congenital agenesis of the gallbladder. A diagnostic problem, *Military Med.*, 150, 283, 1985.
36. **O'Sullivan, J., O'Brien, P. A., MacFeely, L., and Whelton, M. J.,** Congenital absence of the gallbladder and cystic duct: nonoperative diagnosis, *Am. J. Gastroenterol.*, 82, 1190, 1987.
37. **Pinch, L. W.,** Letter to the editor. Agenesis of the gallbladder, *Surgery*, 100, 942, 1986.
38. **James, N. K. and Leaper, D. J.,** Further problems with thalidomide, *J. R. Coll. Surg. Edinburgh*, 34, 167, 1989.
39. **Wilson, J. E. and Deitrick, J. E.,** Agenesis of the gallbladder: case report and familial investigation, *Surgery*, 99, 106, 1986.
40. **Nadeau, L. A., Cloutier, W. A., Konecki, J. T., Morin, G., and Taylor, R. W.,** Hereditary gallbladder agenesis, *J. Maine Med. Assoc.*, 63, 1, 1972.
41. **Kobacher, J. L.** Congenital absence of the gall bladder—a possible hereditary defect, *Ann. Intern. Med.*, 33, 1008, 1950.
42. **Bennion, R. S., Thompson, J. E., and Tompkins, R. K.,** Agenesis of the gallbladder without extrahepatic biliary atresia, *Arch. Surg.*, 123, 1257, 1988.

Chapter 7

VARIATIONS OF FORM

Jon W. Meilstrup and Kenneth D. Hopper

TABLE OF CONTENTS

0-8493-4788-2/94/$0.00+$.50

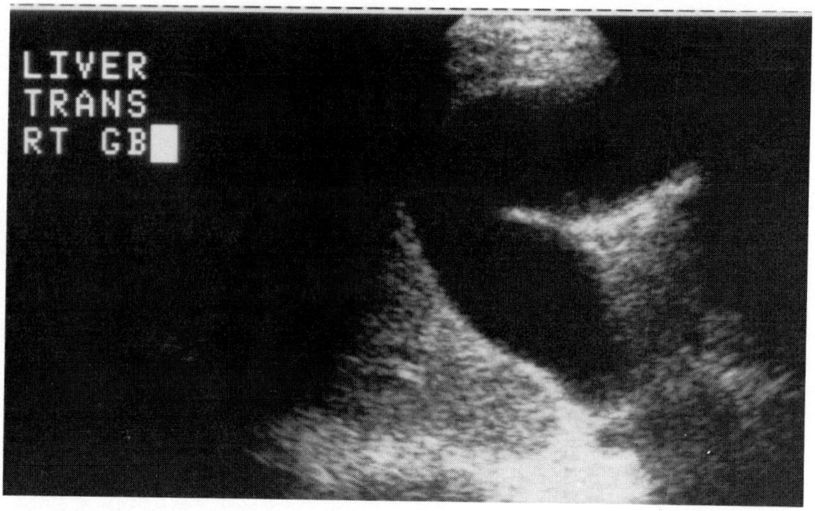

A

FIGURE 1. Sonogram in two different patients (A, B) shows the typical posterior "junctional fold" (arrow). Note cystic duct in B.

I. INTRODUCTION

In 1948 Lockwood[1] classified congenital anomalies of the gallbladder into three basic types: anomalies of location, number, and form. Of these, anomalies of form had the largest number of different subtypes. This category of variants includes various kinds of gallbladder folding (including the Phrygian cap), septations, unusual gallbladder shapes, and the uncommon gallbladder diverticulum, bilobed gallbladder, and rudimentary gallbladder.

II. FOLDING OF THE GALLBLADDER

A. Junctional Fold

Folding of the gallbladder is a frequent finding, occurring in 14.5% of patients.[2] Folds or kinks usually occur in the gallbladder body and have been termed "junctional folds"[3,4] (Figure 1). While they are seen most commonly along the posterior surface, occasionally they are demonstrated anteriorly[5] (Figure 2). A junctional fold appears as a linear filling defect on oral cholecystography or as a dense or echogenic line on computed tomography (CT) (Figure 3) or sonography, respectively. Unlike septations, which are present on all views, gallbladder folds are not constantly seen on all projections. Because they can occasionally cast acoustic shadows, junctional folds may be confused with small calculi or polyps.[3]

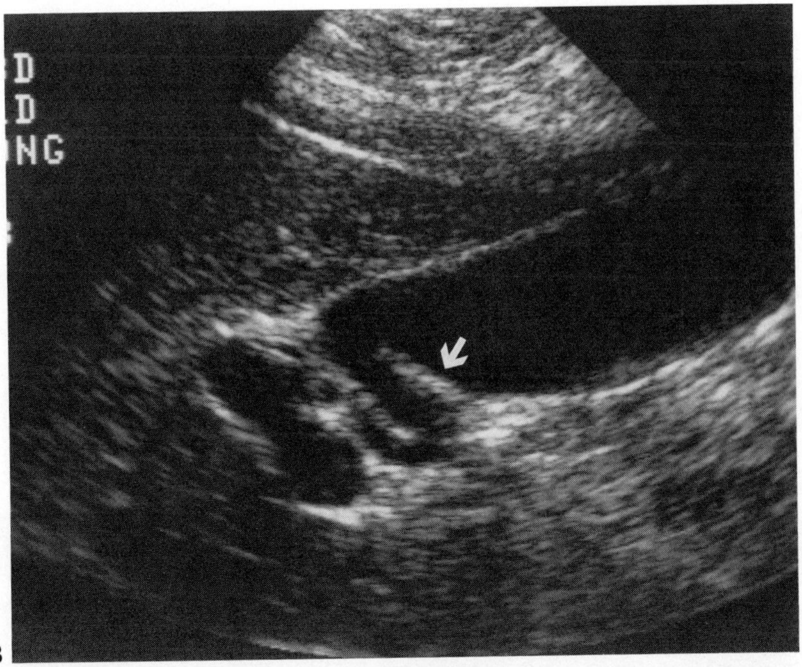

B

FIGURE 1. *Continued.*

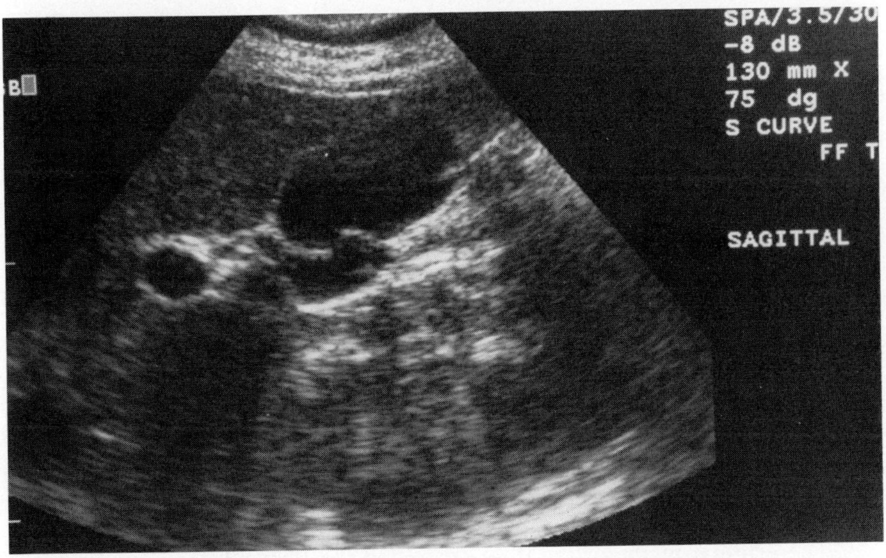

FIGURE 2. Longitudinal sonogram of gallbladder with multiple folds; note the less common anterior fold.

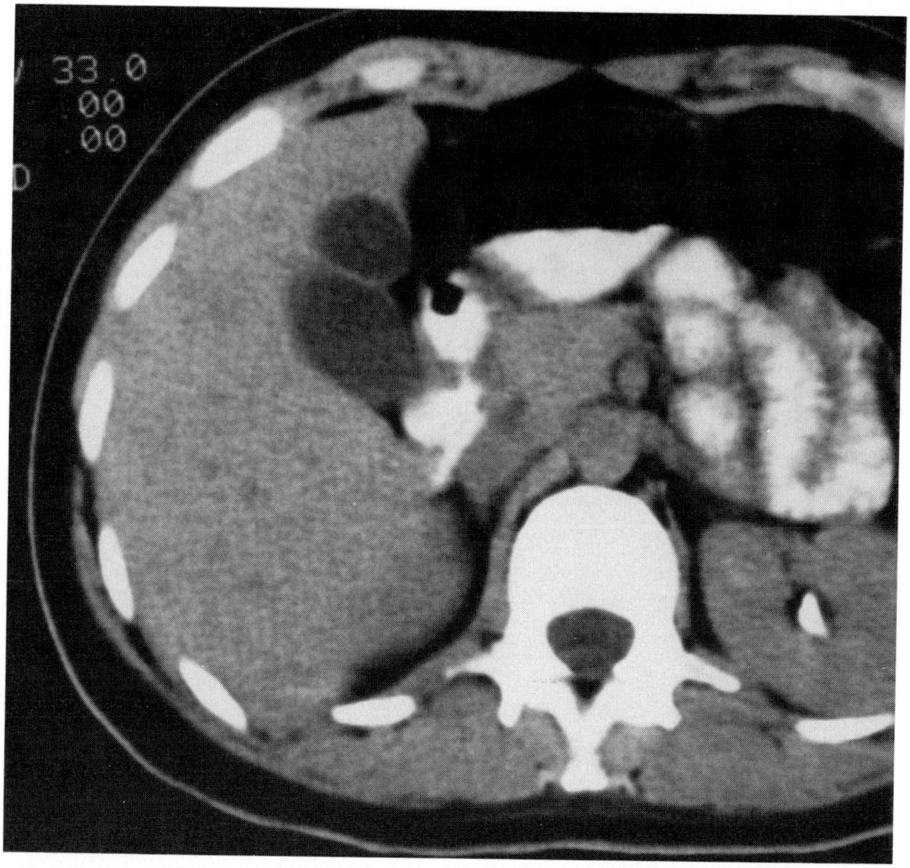

FIGURE 3. CT example of gallbladder fold; this may be difficult to differentiate from a gallbladder septation.

B. Phrygian Cap

The Phrygian cap is a specific type of gallbladder fold. It was originally described with the fundus of the gallbladder being "bent down to the breaking point."[2] This anomaly resembles the Phrygian cap, headgear worn by the ancient Greeks and Romans, and later by French Revolutionary patriots, having the apex folded toward the front.[6] While originally believed to represent disease, the Phrygian cap is now known to be an anomaly of form, and is said to be the most common anomaly of the gallbladder, occurring in about 4% of the general population[6–8] (Figure 4).

The original medical literature described the Phrygian cap as "transitions from a groove to a deep bend caused by a distinctive fold,"[2] which

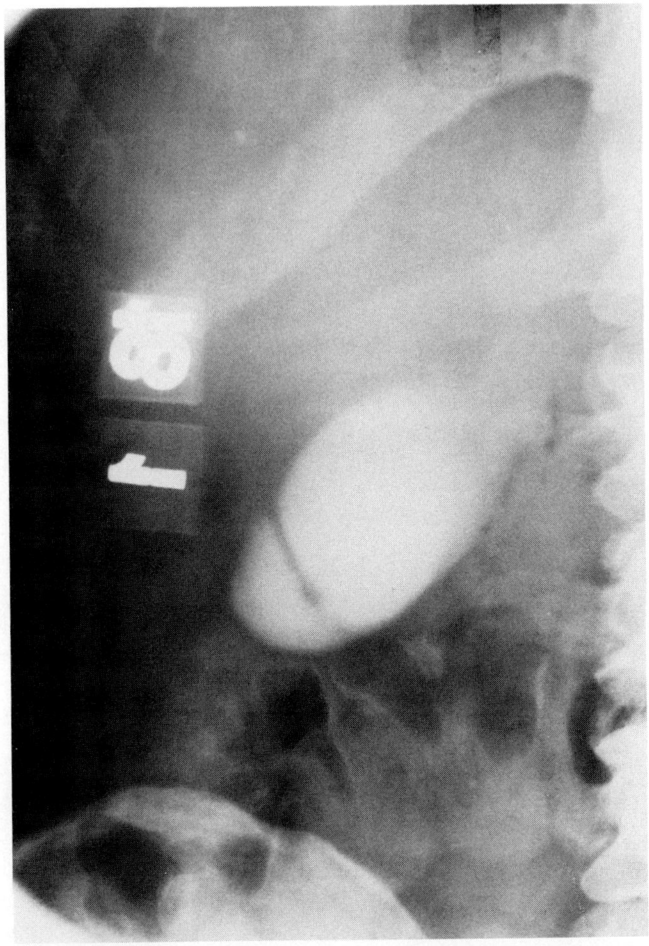

A

FIGURE 4. Examples of Phrygian cap on oral cholecystography (A), sonography (B, C), and CT (D, E). A septation is simulated on (C) by the Phrygian cap seen *en face*. (A, C, and D from Meilstrup, J. W., Hopper, K. D., and Thieme, G. A., *AJR*, 157, 1205, 1991. With permission.)

usually occurred on the medial side of the gallbladder. In 1935 Boyden[2] noted that 18% of 165 patients demonstrated a fold between the body and the infundibulum of the gallbladder or between the body and the fundus. He then classified these folds into two types: a retroserosal or concealed type, which occurs early in development, and a serosal type caused by the attachment of congenital ligaments or septa.[2] Today, any fundal folding variants are generally categorized as Phrygian caps.

This anomaly is of no clinical significance; however, there has been a report of a Phrygian cap with delayed filling on scintigraphy which

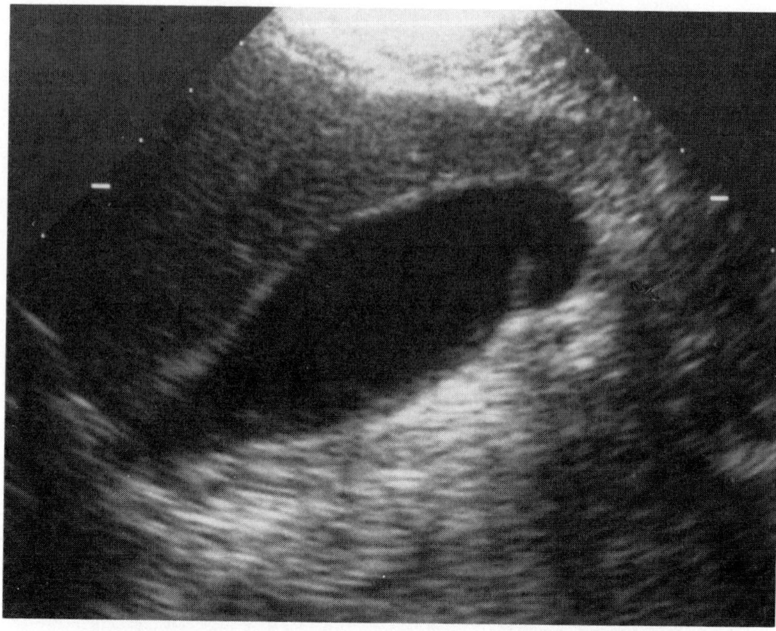

B

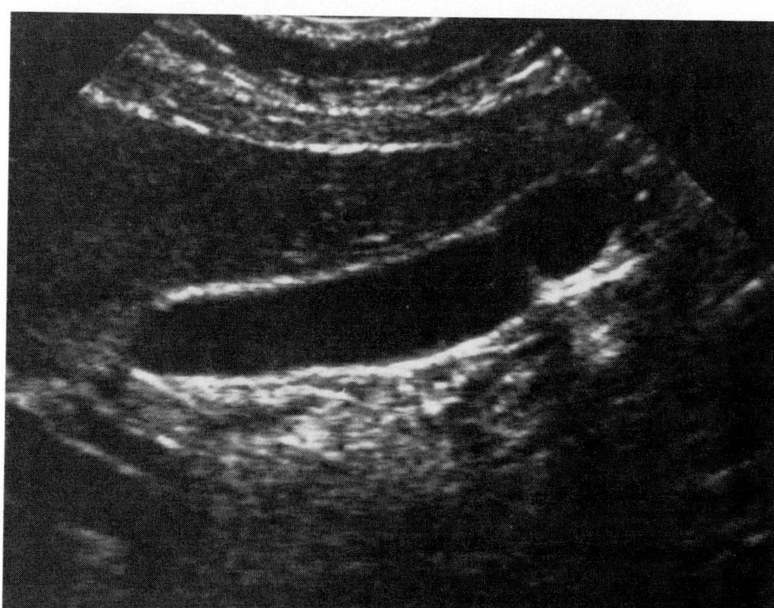

C

FIGURE 4. *Continued.*

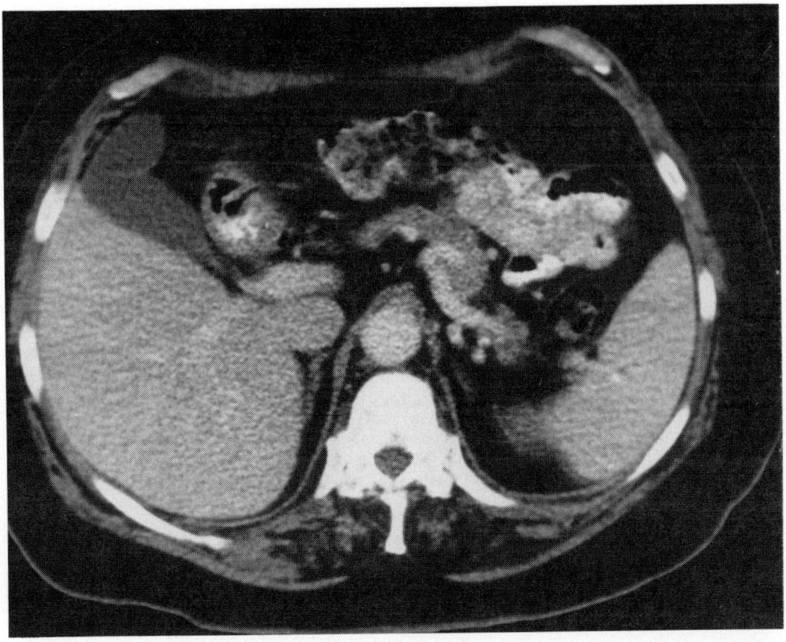

D

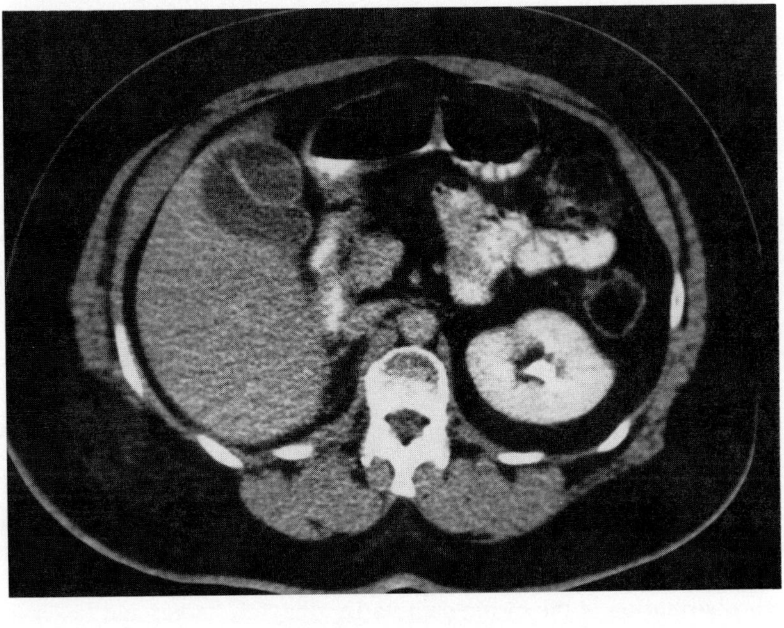

E

FIGURE 4. *Continued.*

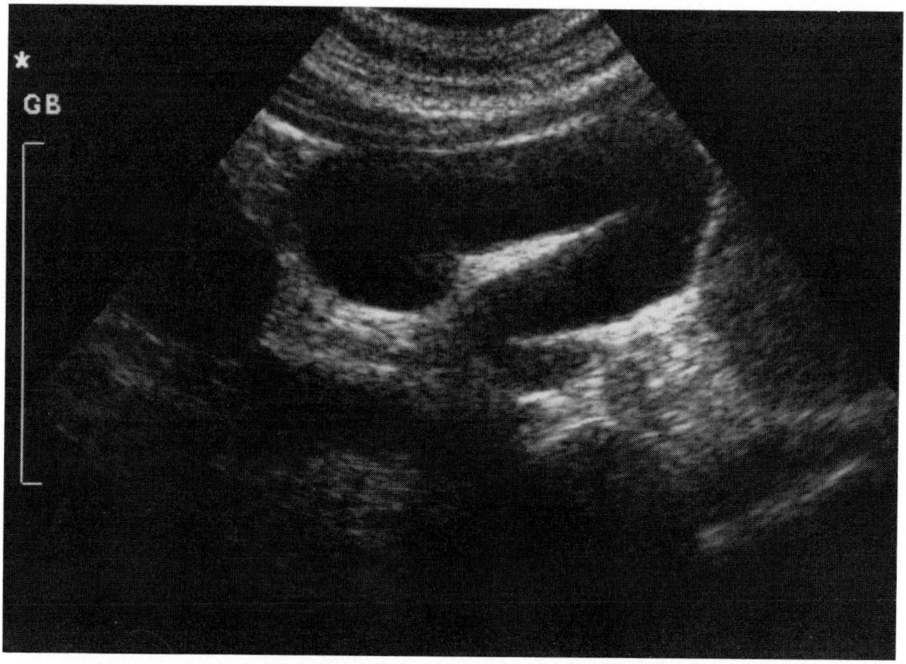

FIGURE 5. Tortuous gallbladder on sonogram.

simulated a mass lesion.[10] A Phrygian cap seen *en face* on oral cholecystography may simulate a mass lesion, but other projections will reveal it as a normal variant.

C. Miscellaneous Folds

Other types of gallbladder folding occur less frequently than the Phrygian cap. Occasionally the gallbladder assumes a very tortuous appearance (Figure 5), such as the ''swan-shaped gallbladder,'' which on some views can simulate a multilocular cyst.[9] A ''boomerang'' gallbladder, with a less tight fold, can mimic a pancreatic pseudocyst on transverse CT images.[5] Like the Phrygian cap, these folds are of no clinical significance.[10]

III. GALLBLADDER NECK AND VALVES OF HEISTER

A dilated common bile duct can be simulated by a tortuous or redundant gallbladder neck. This is generally recognized by careful real-time ultrasound scanning.[11] The valves of Heister are spiral folds or mucous membrane projections that line the cystic duct and gallbladder neck.[3] While their distribution in the cystic duct varies, they are larger and fewer at the distal end, and smaller and more numerous near the junction with the common duct. These valves are arranged in a spiral clockwise fashion and commonly overlap, which may make it difficult to probe the cystic duct at

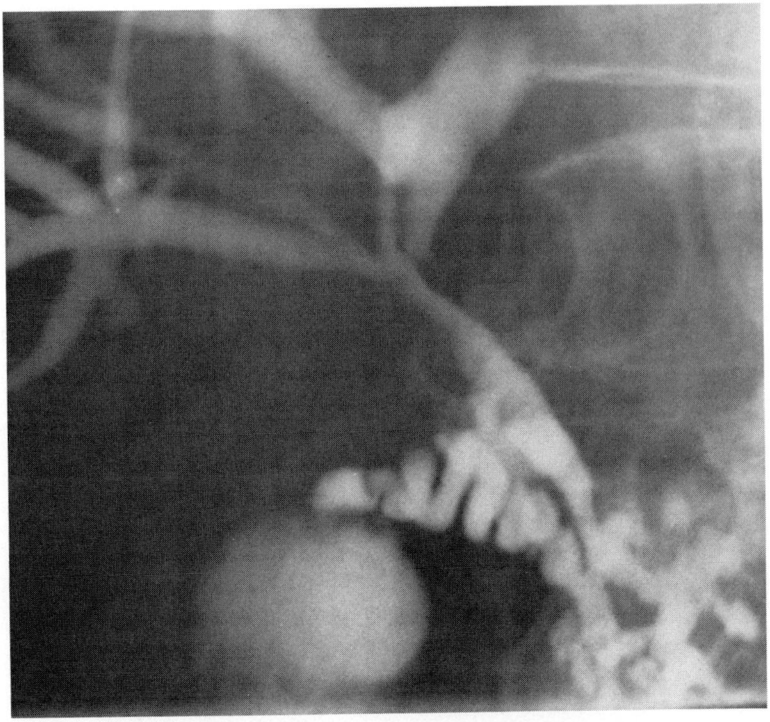
A

FIGURE 6. Valves of Heister on endoscopic retrograde cholecystopancreatography (ERCP) (A), percutaneous transhepatic cholecystography (B), sonography (C, D), and CT (E, F).

surgery. Normally the number of valves range from 1 to 22, although in one series of 308 patients, 8 had no identifiable valves.[12]

Valves of Heister can be readily seen on contrast studies of the gallbladder. They appear as thin, almost linear filling defects on contrast studies (Figure 6A and B). Occasionally, valves of Heister can be seen on sonography and CT (Figure 6C, D, and E).

IV. SEPTATIONS

While small millimeter-sized folds are normal in the gallbladder, true septations are uncommon. Possible etiologies include: (1) a congenital mucosal diaphragm that results from incomplete cannulation of the lumen at development; (2) adenomyomatosis, which develops on a congenital diaphragm, or (3) both.[13] Gallbladder septations may be partial or complete (Figure 7), can cause bile stasis, and may be associated with inflammation and cholelithiasis. Septations are often multiple, ranging from one to three, but a true multiseptate gallbladder is rare.

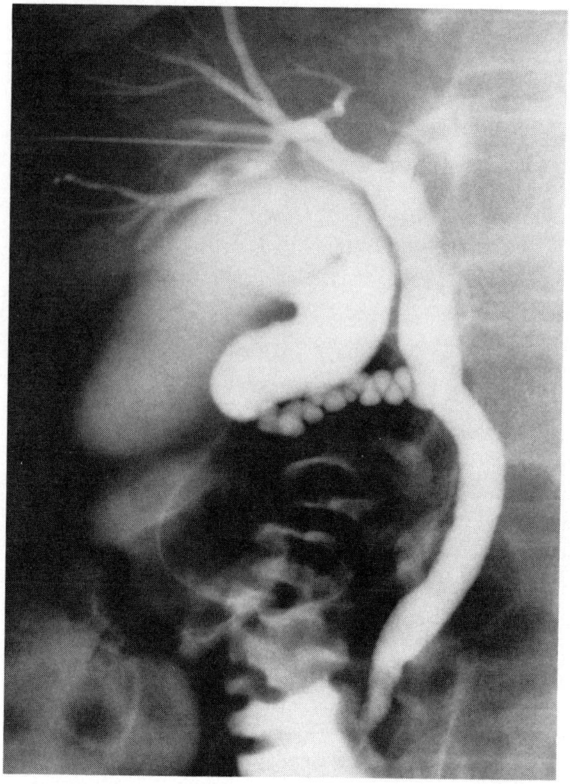

B

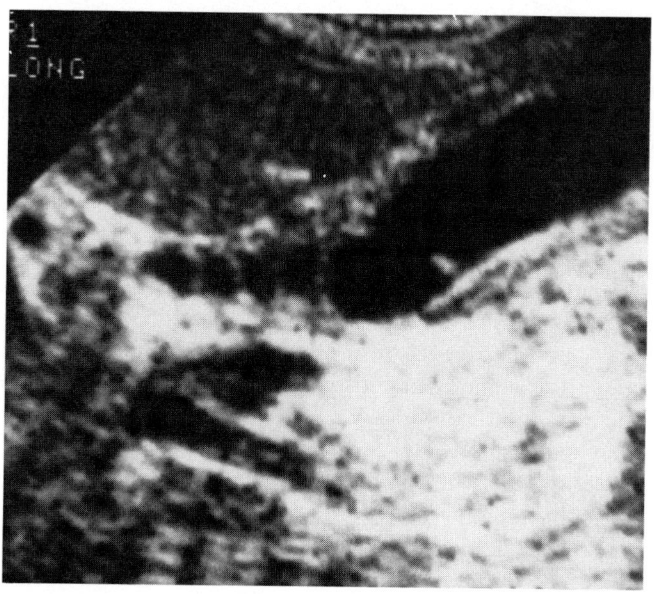

C

FIGURE 6. *Continued.*

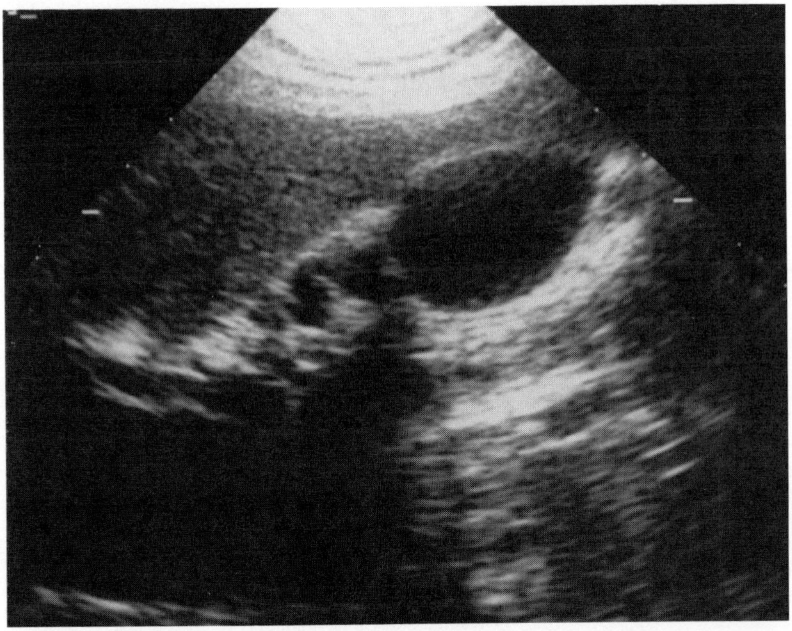

D

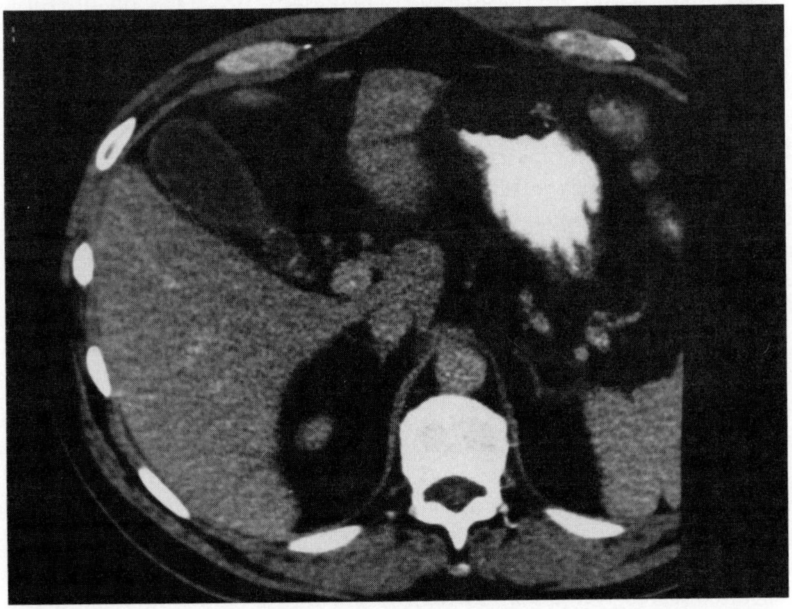

E

FIGURE 6. *Continued.*

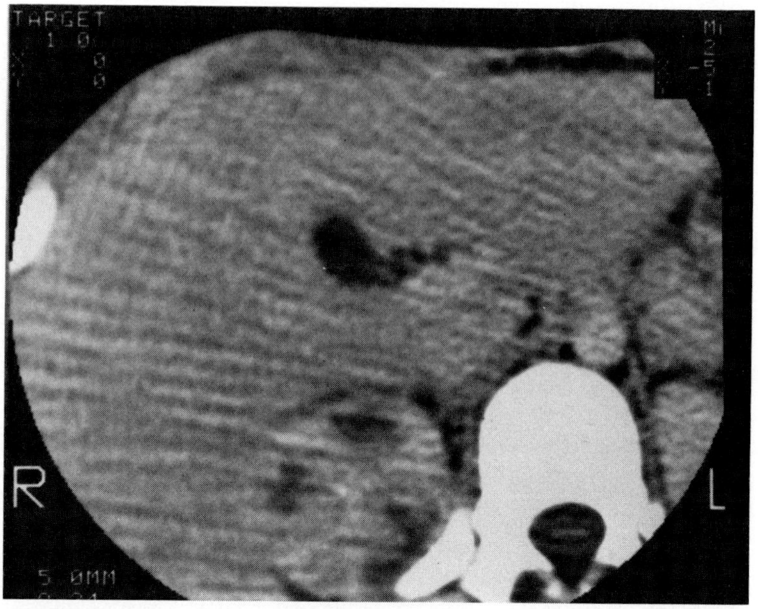

F

FIGURE 6. *Continued.*

Two main septal orientations have been described. The bicameral gallbladder results when a horizontal septation bisects the gallbladder into two chambers, fundal and ductal.[14,27] Longitudinal septation, however, bisects the gallbladder lengthwise. The latter septations are generally included in the spectrum of gallbladder duplication,[15] however, and have been discussed previously (Chapter 6).

On contrast studies a thin isthmus is usually identified between the two compartments. A septated gallbladder also should be suspected on oral cholecystography when a ''flattened fundus'' is seen. This sign occurs because the fundal compartment does not fill, producing a ''flat'' edge of the unopacified compartment.[13] Occasionally a gallbladder septation can mimic a stone by causing a nondependent lucency surrounded by a dense rim of contrast on oral cholecystography or CT.[16] Sonographically, a septation normally appears as an echogenic band (Figure 7C and D). Rarely it can cause edge-shadowing, which could be confused with a stone. In every modality, the septation should be visualized on two right angle views to help distinguish it from a fold.

A. Multiseptate Gallbladder

Multiseptate gallbladder is one of the rarest gallbladder anomalies,[17] with the first detailed case description in 1963.[18] While the exact cause is not known,[19] it is felt to be a congenital anomaly, with its appearance possibly ''resulting from incomplete cavitation of the developing gallbladder bud. The lumen . . . remains divided by many septa, formed by the mucosal, submucosal, and muscular layers extending from the outer wall.''[18]

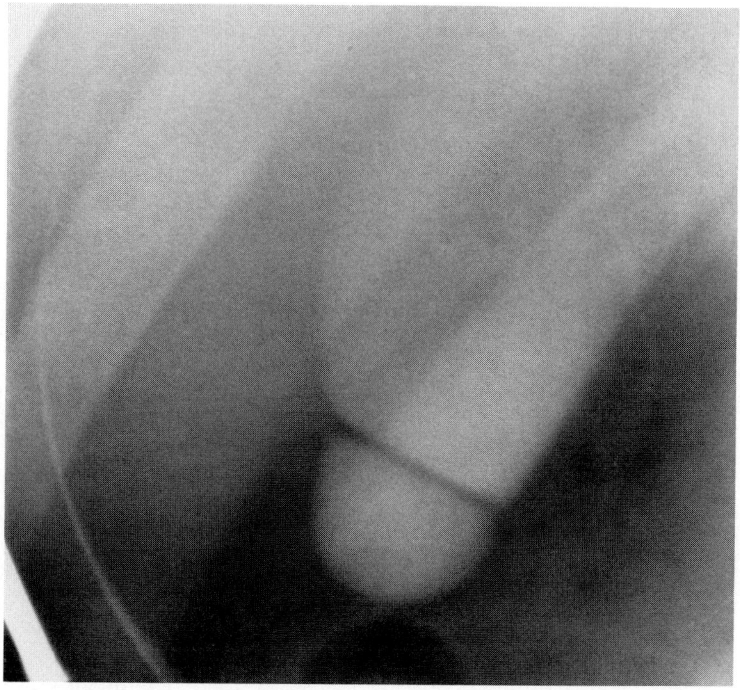

A

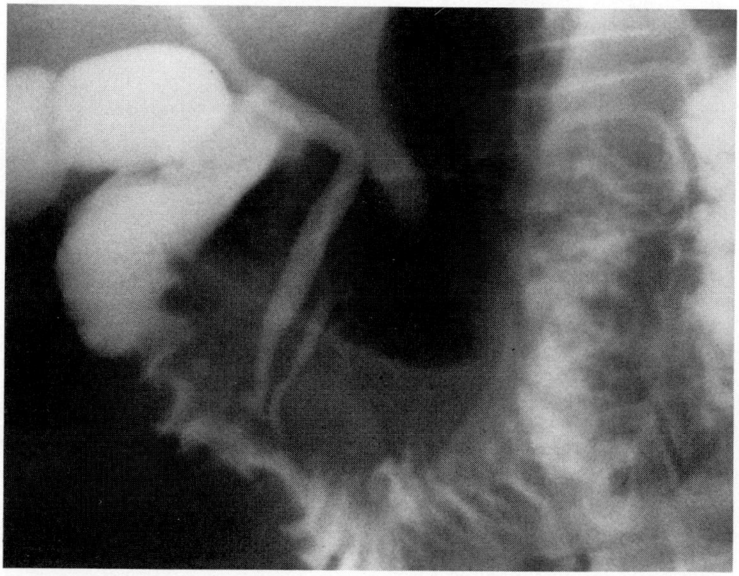

B

FIGURE 7. Examples of septation on oral cholecystography (A), ERCP (B), sonography (C, D), and CT (E). (D) and (E) are partial septations. (B, C, and D from Meilstrup, J. W., Hopper, K. D., and Thieme, G. A., *AJR,* 157, 1205, 1991. With permission.)

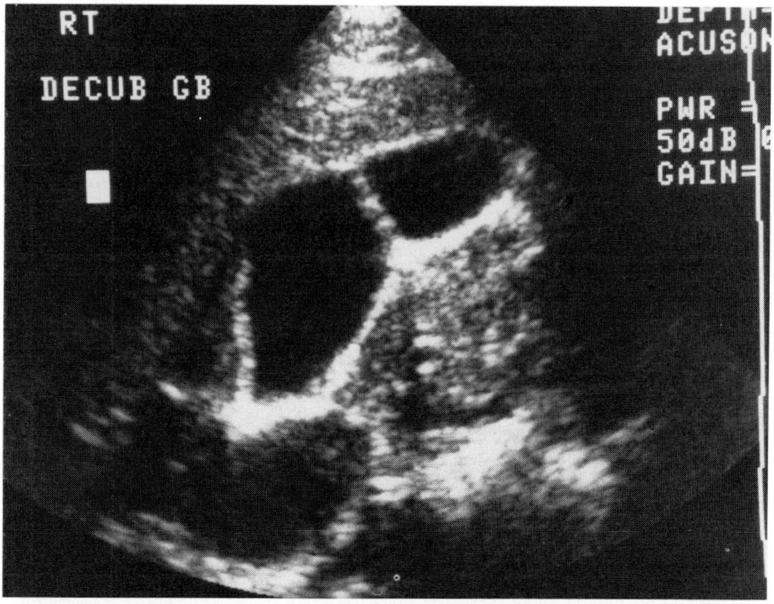

C

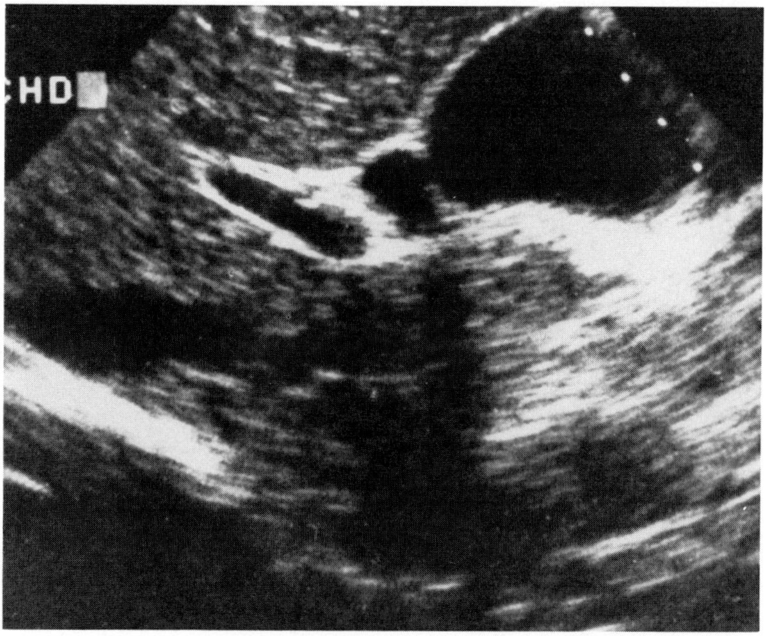

D

FIGURE 7. *Continued.*

E 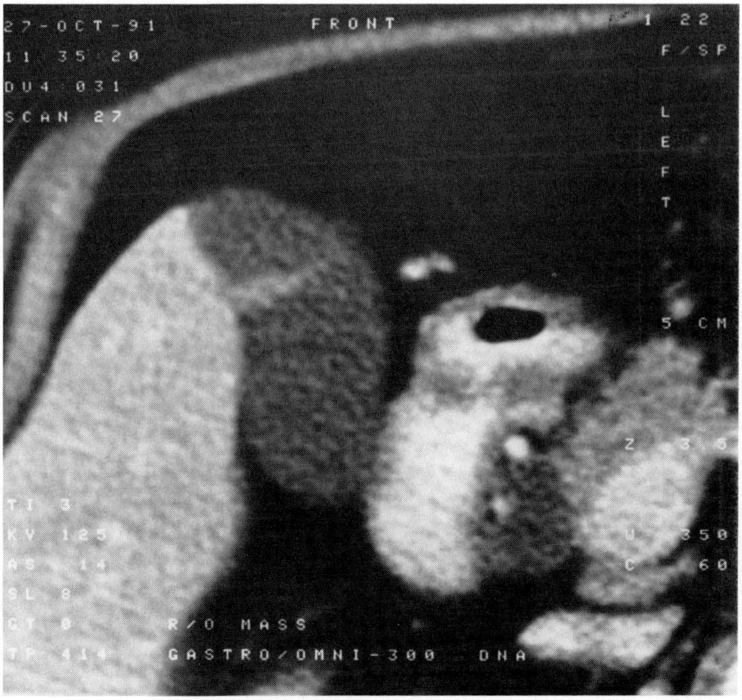

FIGURE 7. *Continued.*

These resulting small compartments intercommunicate.[18] Another hypothesis contends that a multiseptate gallbladder is due to persistent ''wrinkling'' of the wall associated with cleft formation and lobulation.[20] Emptying of a multiseptate gallbladder may be slower than normal.[18] Associated abdominal symptoms may be seen, although there may be no symptoms and normal gallbladder function.[17,19]

Externally the surface of a multiseptate gallbladder usually appears to be ''faintly bosselated'',[21] having multiple small eminences. The internal septations have a layer of muscle that is situated between two epithelial layers.[21,22] These septations are irregular and ''run in all directions''.[19] This pattern has been described at different times as a honeycomb, mosaic, trabeculated, or multilocular pattern.[17-24] The multiseptate gallbladder may be normal in size.[25]

Sonographic reports of multiseptate gallbladder are uncommon;[17,23,26] most reported cases have been demonstrated by oral cholecystography, but sonography can demonstrate this entity well (Figure 8). The major sonographic features are described as ''multiple fine, non-shadowing septations that bridge the gallbladder lumen.''[17] Multiseptate changes may rarely involve only a part of the gallbladder (the ''partial multiseptate gall-

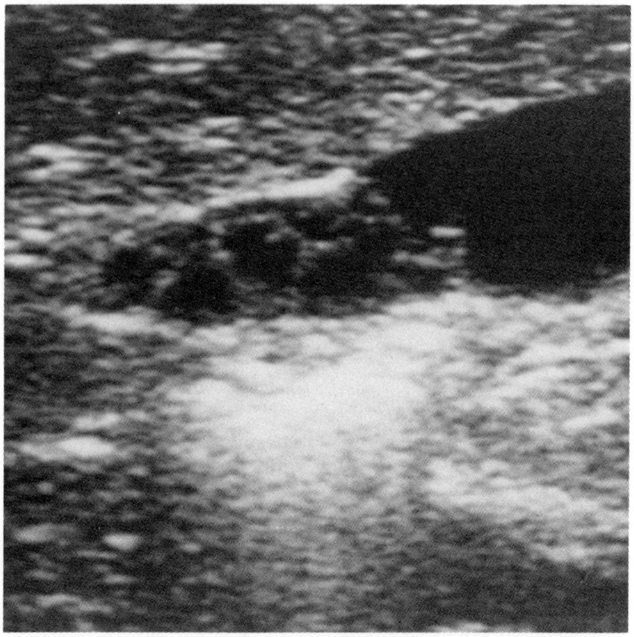

A

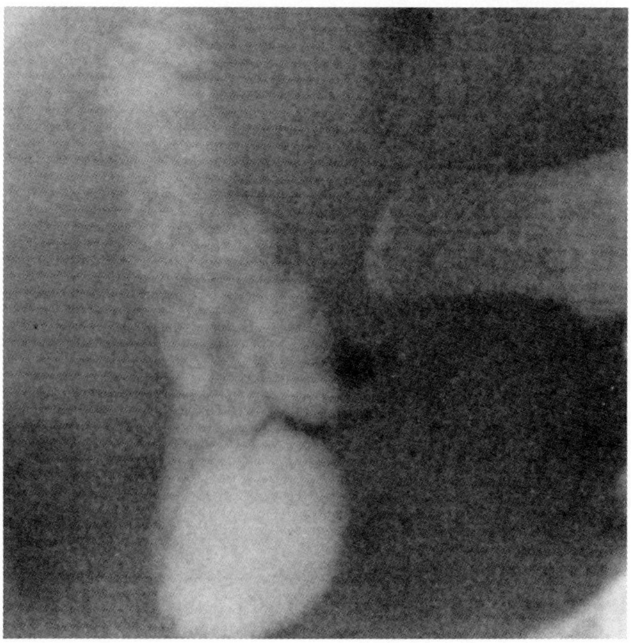

B

FIGURE 8. Multiseptate gallbladder. This is a rare anomaly, with multiple septations, giving a "honeycomb" appearance on longitudinal sonography (A) and oral cholecystogram (B). (C) Coronal sonogram of another patient. (A, B, and C from Lev-Toaff, A. S., Friedman, A. C., Rindsberg, S. N., Caroline, D. F., Maurer, A. H., and Radecki, P. D., *AJR,* 148, 1119, 1987. With permission.)

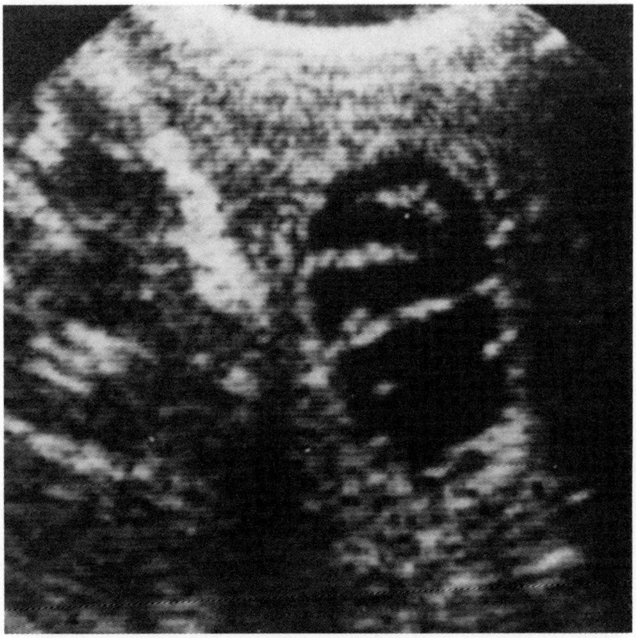

C

FIGURE 8. *Continued.*

bladder'').[27] On imaging, differential diagnostic considerations include hyperplastic cholecystoses, desquamated gallbladder mucosa, and possibly adenomyomatosis.[17,26]

V. MISCELLANEOUS

The so-called hourglass gallbladder represents a type of bilobed gallbladder. A transverse septum or stricture divides the body and infundibulum, creating two compartments. This anomaly is also referred to as a compartmental gallbladder or stricture of the gallbladder (Figure 9). This configuration can be acquired or congenital.[15,28,29] Fewer than 1% of patients demonstrate this anomaly, which predisposes to cholelithiasis.

Gallbladder diverticula are rare. They can be found anywhere in the gallbladder, arising from persistent cystohepatic ducts or their remnants which open directly into the gallbladder.[28] While these diverticula may be asymptomatic, they can be associated with bile stasis and accompanying inflammatory changes and stone disease. Like other diverticula, they can also perforate.

Ducts of Luschka[30] are structurally the same as intrahepatic bile ducts, and occasionally are found on the hepatic surface of gallbladder wall specimens. Ducts of Luschka are different from Rokitansky-Aschoff sinuses, which are small intramural diverticula, crypts, or sinus tracts,[31] while ducts

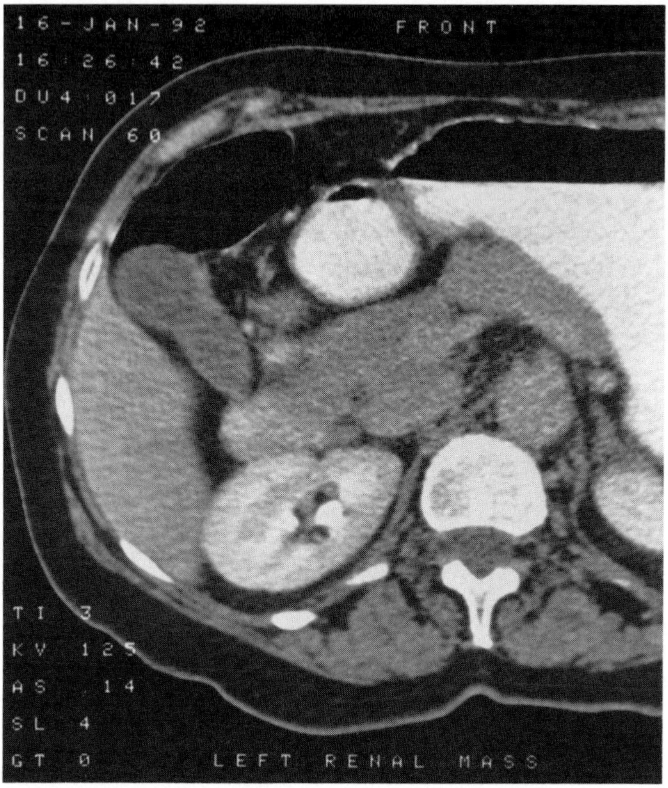

FIGURE 9. Hourglass gallbladder seen on CT examination of a 61-year-old female.

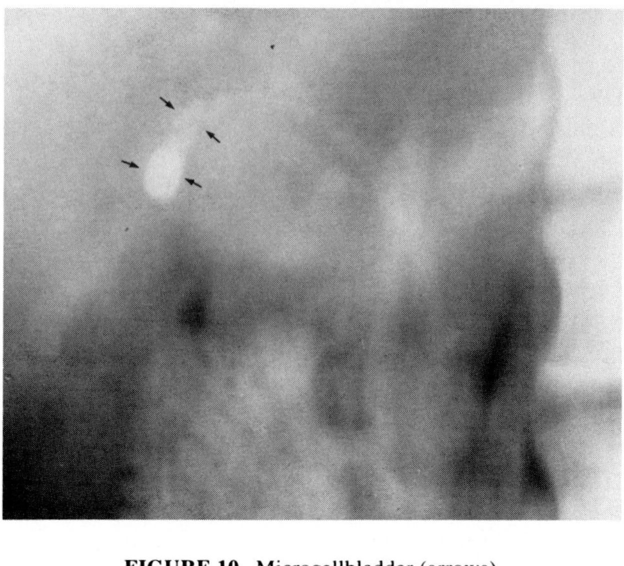

FIGURE 10. Microgallbladder (arrows).

of Luschka have not been visualized on imaging studies, Rokitansky-Aschoff sinuses can be seen on oral cholecystography, CT, and occasionally sonography.

The normal adult gallbladder is variable in size, measuring from 7 to 10 cm in length and 2 to 4 cm in width.[32,33] A giant, congenitally enlarged gallbladder has been described, measuring up to 18 cm in length.[34] Rarely is a small or rudimentary gallbladder (microgallbladder) imaged (Figure 10). When identified in children it probably represents the result of congenital hypoplasia. However, a microgallbladder in adults may be postinflammatory.[27] Micro- and macrogallbladders may also be seen in cystic fibrosis.[35–37] A multiseptate microgallbladder has been reported as a rare combination of two anomalies.[38]

REFERENCES

1. **Lockwood, B. C.,** Congenital anomalies of the gallbladder, *JAMA,* 10, 678, 1948.
2. **Boyden, E. A.,** The "Phrygian cap" in cholecystography. A congenital anomaly of the gallbladder, *Am. J. Roentgenol. Rad. Ther.,* 33, 589, 1935.
3. **Sukov, R. J., Sample, W. F., Sarti, D. A., and Whitcomb, M. J.,** Cholecystosonography—the junctional fold, *Radiology,* 133, 435, 1979.
4. **Grant, J. C. B.,** *An Atlas of Anatomy,* Williams & Wilkins, Baltimore, 1972, 161.
5. **Meilstrup, J. W., Hopper, K. D., and Thieme, G. A.,** Imaging of gallbladder variants, *AJR,* 157, 1205, 1991.
6. **Ober, W. B. and Wharton, R. N.,** On the "Phrygian cap", *N. Engl. J. Med.,* 255, 571, 1956.
7. **Meyer, W. H., Carter, R. F., and Meeker, L. H.,** The "Phrygian cap" deformity of the gallbladder, *AJR,* 37, 786, 1937.
8. **Edell, S.,** A comparison of the "Phrygian cap" deformity with bistable and gray scale ultrasound, *J. Clin. Ultrasound,* 6, 34, 1978.
9. **Morcos, S. K.,** Letter to the editor. The swan-shaped gallbladder, *J. Clin. Ultrasound,* 13, 299, 1985.
10. **Smergel, E. M. and Maurer, A. H.,** Phrygian cap simulating mass lesion in hepatobiliary scintigraphy, *Clin. Nucl. Med.,* 9, 131, 1984.
11. **Laing, F. C. and Jeffrey, R. B.,** The pseudo-dilated common bile duct: ultrasonographic appearance created by the gallbladder neck, *Radiology,* 135, 405, 1980.
12. **Mentzer, S. H.,** The valves of Heister, *Arch. Surg.,* 13, 511, 1926.
13. **Doyle, T. C.,** Flattened fundus sign of the septate gallbladder, *Gastrointest. Radiol.,* 9, 345, 1984.
14. **Murayama, S., Mizyshima, A., Russell, W. J., and Higashi, Y.,** Sonographic diagnosis of bicameral gallbladders: a report of three cases, *J. Ultrasound Med.,* 4, 539, 1985.
15. **Blumberg, N. A.,** Transverse septum of the gallbladder, *S. Afr. J. Surg.,* 19, 139, 1981.
16. **Bova, J. G.,** Gallstone simulated by gallbladder septation, *AJR,* 140, 287, 1983.
17. **Lev-Toaff, A. S., Friedman, A. C., Rindsberg, S. N., Caroline, D. F., Maurer, A. H., and Radecki, P. D.,** Multiseptate gallbladder: incidental diagnosis on sonography, *AJR,* 148, 1119, 1987.

18. **Simon, M. and Tandon, B. N.,** Multiseptate gallbladder, *Radiology*, 80, 84, 1963.
19. **Okuda, K., Nakajima, M., Nakayama, M., and Nomura, F.,** Multiseptate gallbladder. Report of a case with a review of literature, *Acta Hepato-Gastroenterol.*, 26, 70, 1979.
20. **Bhagavan, B. S., Amin, P. B., Land, A. S., and Weinberg, T.,** Multiseptate gallbladder. Embryogenetic hypotheses, *Arch. Pathol.*, 89, 382, 1970.
21. **Croce, E. J.,** The multiseptate gallbladder, *Arch. Surg.*, 107, 104, 1973.
22. **Toombs, B. D., Foucar, E., Rowlands, B. J., and Strax, R.,** Multiseptate gallbladder, *South. Med. J.*, 75, 610, 1982.
23. **Pery, M., Kaftori, J. K., Marvan, H., Sweed, Y., and Kerner, H.,** Ultrasonographic appearance of multiseptate gallbladder: report of a case with coexisting choledochal cyst, *J. Clin. Ultrasound*, 13, 570, 1985.
24. **Vasinrapee, P., Linden, K., and Cook, R.E.,** Multiseptate gallbladder demonstrated on Tc-99m hepatobiliary imaging, *Clin. Nucl. Med.*, 15, 272, 1990.
25. **Oliva, I. O., Moran, M. R., Sanchez, F. L., and Alonso, A. G.,** Multiseptate gallbladder, *Int. Surg.*, 70, 83, 1985.
26. **Adear, H. and Barki, Y.,** Multiseptate gallbladder in a child: incidental diagnosis on sonography, *Pediatr. Radiol.*, 20, 192, 1990.
27. **Strauss, S., Starinsky, R., and Alon, Z.,** Partial multiseptate gallbladder: sonographic appearance, *J. Ultrasound Med.*, 4, 201, 1993.
28. **Pontes, J. F. and Pinotti, H. W.,** Anomalies of the gallbladder and biliary system, in *Gastroenterology*, Vol. 3, Bockus, H. L., Ed., W. B. Saunders, Philadelphia, 1976, 651.
29. **Hughes, J. H.,** Hourglass gallbladder: an update, *Military Med.*, 151, 603, 1986.
30. **Robertson, H. E. and Ferguson, W. J.,** The diverticula (Luschka's crypts) of the gallbladder, *Arch. Pathol.*, 40, 312, 1945.
31. **Berk, R. N., van der Vegt, J. H., and Lichtenstein, J. E.,** The hyperplastic cholecystoses: cholesterolosis and adenomyomatosis, *Radiology*, 146, 593, 1983.
32. **Mittelstaedt, C. A.,** Biliary system, in *General Ultrasound*, Mittelstaedt, C. A., Ed., Churchill Livingstone, New York, 1992, chap. 6.
33. **McGahan, J. P., Phillips, H. E., and Cox, K. L.,** Sonography of the normal pediatric gallbladder and biliary tract, *Radiology*, 144, 873, 1982.
34. **Maeda, Y., Setoguchi, T., Yoshida, T., and Katsuki, T.,** A giant gallbladder, *Gastroenterol. Jpn.*, 14, 622, 1979.
35. **Hammond, D. I.,** Unusual causes of sonographic nonvisualization or nonrecognition of the gallbladder: a review, *J. Clin. Ultrasound*, 16, 77, 1988.
36. **Lechtonen, L., Svedström, E., and Kervennanta, H.,** The size and contractibility of the gallbladder in infants, *Pediatr. Radiol.*, 22, 515, 1992.
37. **Isdale, J. M., Reef, I., and Pettifor, J. M.,** Gallbladder anomalies and cystic fibrosis, *S. Afr. Med. J.*, 62, 160, 1982.
38. **Jena, P. K., Hardie, R. A., and Hobsley, M.,** Multiseptate hypoplastic gallbladder, *Br. J. Surg.*, 64, 192, 1977.

Chapter 8

ARTIFACTS

Claudia J. Kasales, Gary A. Thieme, and Jon W. Meilstrup

The development of cross-sectional imaging studies such as sonography, computed tomography (CT), and magnetic resonance imaging (MRI) has dramatically changed the clinical workup of gallbladder disease. Each imaging modality, however, is subject to several potential physical artifacts that are characteristic of that modality. Some, such as sound attenuation and acoustic enhancement, are useful. Other artifacts such as refraction and off-axis energy, however, can mimic the presence of disease.[1,2] Familiarity with the appearance and origins of artifacts affecting the normal gallbladder allows more accurate assessment, avoiding the potential for misdiagnosis.

Ultrasound imaging quality is influenced by several parameters. Intrinsic factors such as the patient body habitus and the acoustic impedance of the organ system being studied cannot be changed. However, extrinsic factors such as the type of transducer utilized (Figure 1), the scanning frequency (Figure 2), the acoustic window, and the system control settings are more

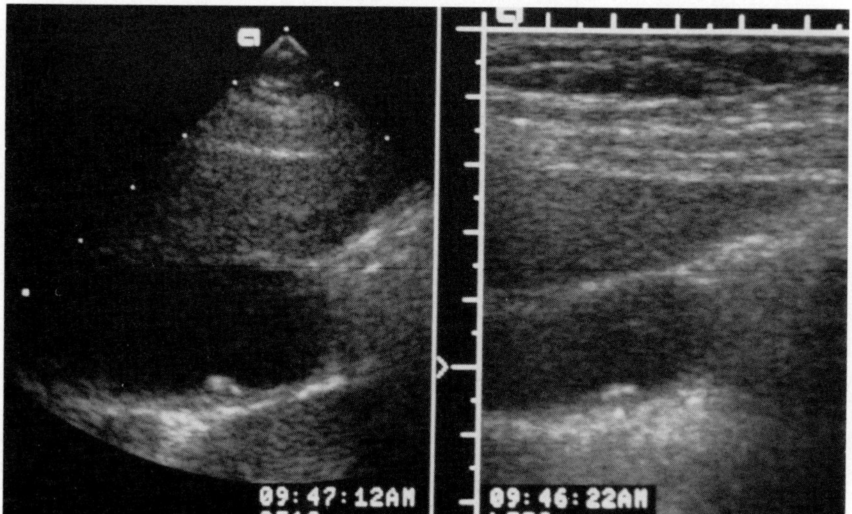

FIGURE 1. The narrow footprint of the sector transducer provides a clear image of the gallbladder (A). With the wide footprint of the linear array transducer, noise from scattered sound energy obscures image detail (B).

0-8493-4788-2/94/$0.00+$.50

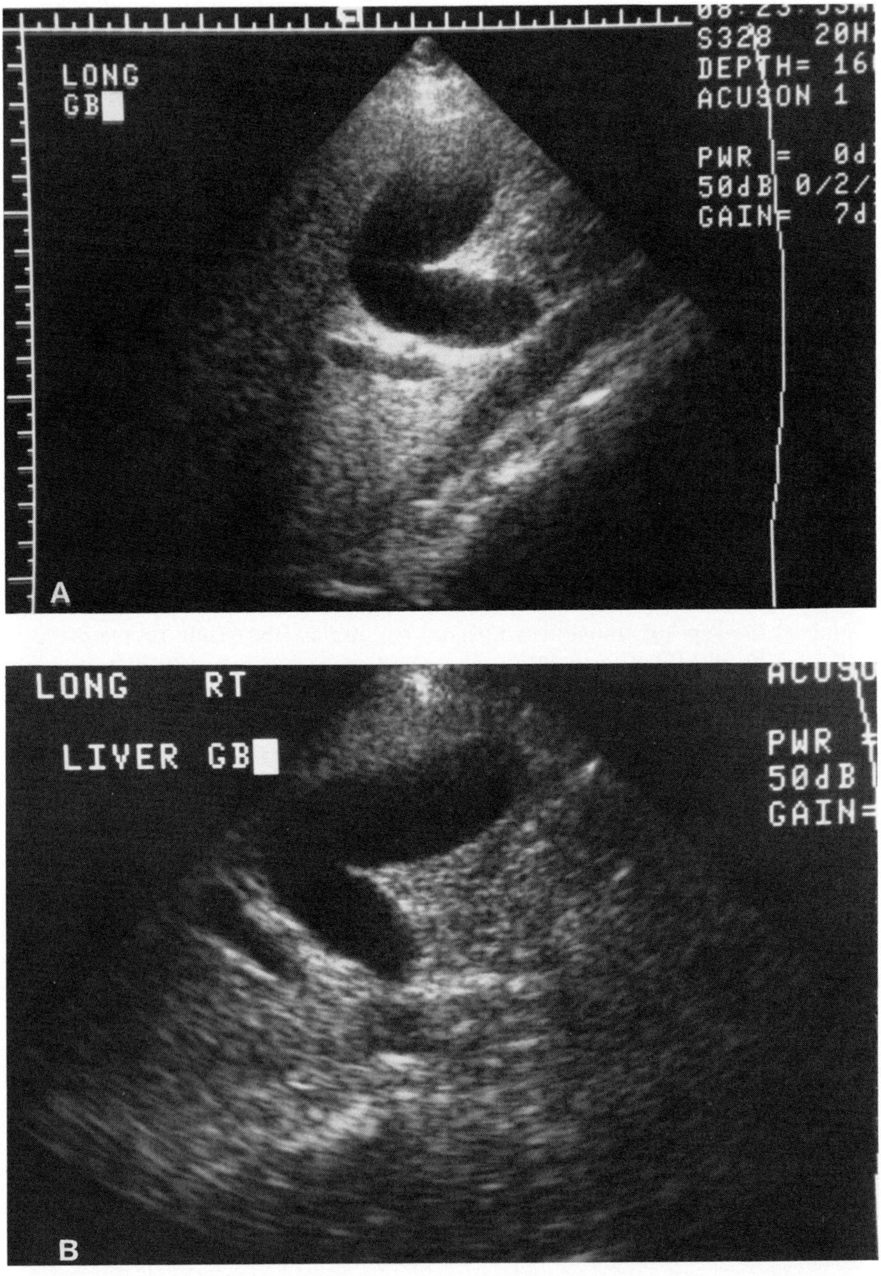

FIGURE 2. Longitudinal sonograms obtained with (A) 3 MHz and (B) 2.25 MHz transducers. While higher frequency transducers often produce the best images, this must be optimized for each patient. In some cases, the gallbladder may be better seen with the improved penetration obtained by lower frequency transducers, as in (B). Note C-shaped gallbladder with a prominent junctional fold.

readily varied and can have a strong impact on image quality.[3] Although general guidelines are useful, the scanning process remains operator dependent, and scanning experience is the most important factor in obtaining high-quality studies.

Spatial resolution in ultrasound is determined by both the frequency and focusing properties of the transducer. Resolution is better at higher scanning frequencies because the shorter sound wavelength provides better axial resolution and enables sharper focusing, reducing partial volume artifact. However, higher frequency transducers are limited by the depth of sound penetration, which is inversely related to the scanning frequency.

Equally important with respect to spatial resolution are the electronic focusing properties of modern linear array and sector array transducers, which allow the user to select the depth of focus in the X–Y plane. Electronic focusing concentrates sound energy into a narrow beam at the level of interest, reducing or eliminating artifacts associated with partial volume averaging. The depth of focus in the slice-thickness (Z axis) plane, however, is fixed by the shape of the acoustic lens and cannot be varied by the user. Fortunately, X–Y plane focusing effects dominate Z axis focusing effects making selection of a transducer with the proper slice-thickness plane focusing less critical. By contrast, annular array transducers have a symmetrically focused beam and do not suffer the same degradation in Z axis resolution as linear and sector array transducers.

In gallbladder imaging, the optimization of scanning frequency and focusing properties is highly dependent upon patient body habitus. For thin adults and children 5 and 7.5 MHz scanning frequencies are optimal. Average adults are often best imaged with 3.5 and 5 MHz transducers, while imaging the gallbladder in large adults or obese patients may require the use of a 2.25-MHz transducer. Despite reduced spatial resolution, the deeper penetration and the reduction of imaging artifacts afforded by lower frequency transducers often result in better image quality when compared with higher frequency transducers (Figure 2). Intraoperative imaging of the gallbladder, on the other hand, is not limited by patient habitus and can usually be achieved with a 10-MHz transducer.

Reflection and refraction artifacts[4,5] are commonly encountered in gallbladder sonography. The multiple reflective paths within the layers of the abdominal wall can cause reverberation artifacts. Such artifacts can be seen as either a distinct band or a diffuse haze of echoes within the gallbladder lumen, mimicking sludge (Figure 3). Recognizing that reverberation echo amplitude usually decreases with increasing distance from the transducer can help verify its artifactual nature. Generally, artifacts are not consistently reproducible during real time scanning and changing the acoustic window frequently will clear the echoes from the gallbladder lumen.

Refraction artifacts often occur at the edges of rounded structures whose acoustic impedance differs from that of the surrounding medium. The lens effect of the curved surfaces being imaged (such as the gallbladder wall)

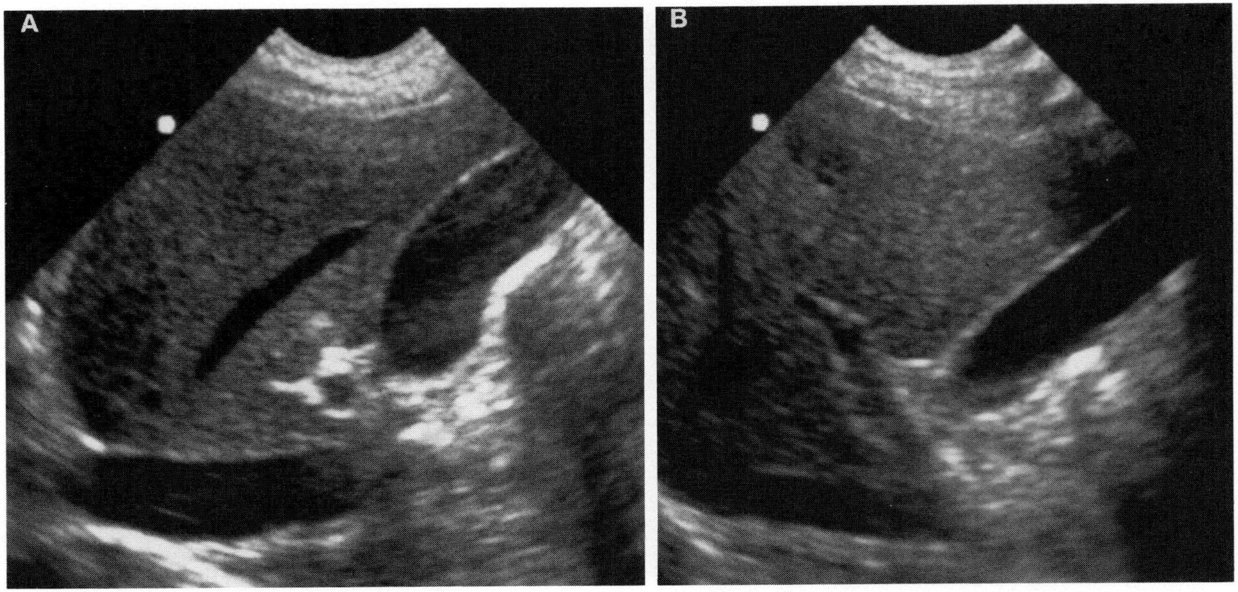

FIGURE 3. Reverberation artifacts from the abdominal wall obscure the lumen of the gallbladder (A, left). Changing the acoustic window eliminates the artifactual echoes from reverberation (B, right), although side-lobe artifact can still be seen.

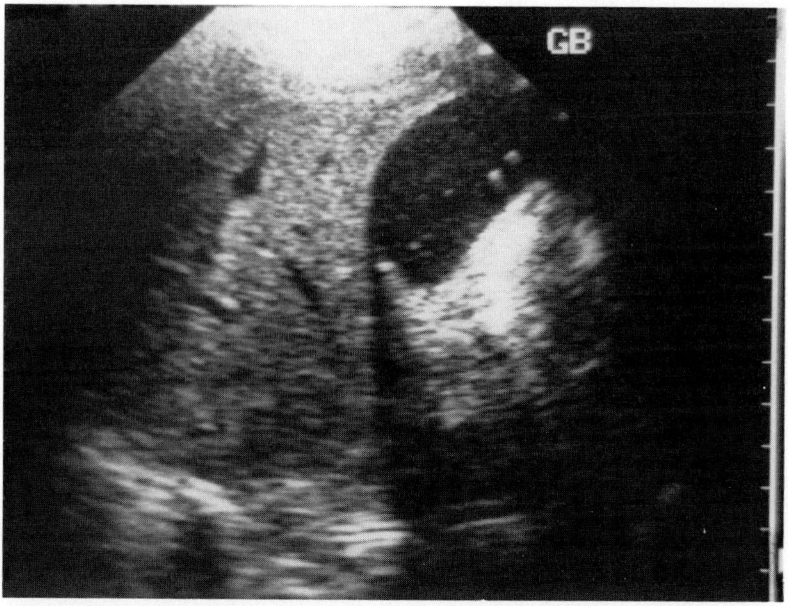

FIGURE 4. A critical angle refractory shadow at the margin of the gallbladder with the liver should not be mistaken for a stone in the neck. The gallbladder is full of sludge, with several punctate nonshadowing densities also seen in the gallbladder lumen.

can cause the sound beam to be bent away from a straight-line path when the beam is nearly tangential to the interface. Because sound energy cannot return to the transducer from points beyond the usual straight-line path, a narrow region devoid of echoes is produced, resembling an acoustic shadow. This artifact is commonly seen along the margins of the gallbladder and can mimic the shadow from a gallstone.[5] However, no echogenic focus can be identified as the source of the shadow, enabling the observer to differentiate this artifact from a true calculus. Altering the scan angle will usually eliminate the artifact (Figure 4).

The rounded shape of the gallbladder and its cystic nature predispose it to side-lobe or grating-lobe artifacts.[6] Transducer side lobes and grating lobes produce a cone of low intensity sound energy centered around the main axis of the ultrasound beam. This off-axis sound energy generally is of little consequence when scanning. However, when it returns to the transducer from highly reflective surfaces (such as bowel gas) adjacent to the gallbladder, the ultrasound system projects this received off-axis energy as if it occurred along the central beam axis and produces a radial band of intraluminal echoes which appear to originate from within the gallbladder itself (Figure 5A). If these echoes occur along the dependent gallbladder surface, they may mimic sludge[6] (Figure 5B). Unlike true sludge, however, the surface of this artifact is usually curved and is not gravity dependent.

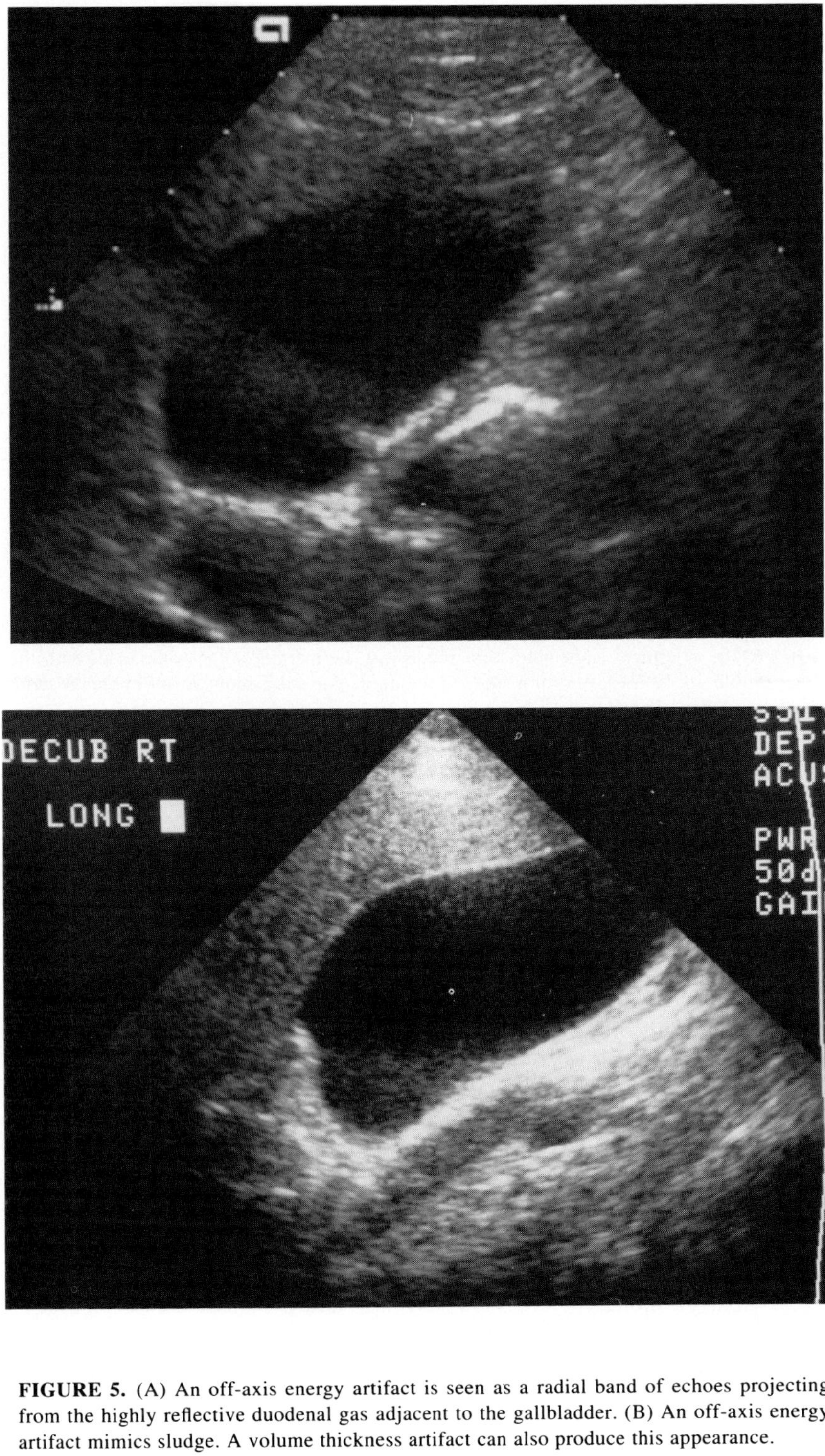

FIGURE 5. (A) An off-axis energy artifact is seen as a radial band of echoes projecting from the highly reflective duodenal gas adjacent to the gallbladder. (B) An off-axis energy artifact mimics sludge. A volume thickness artifact can also produce this appearance.

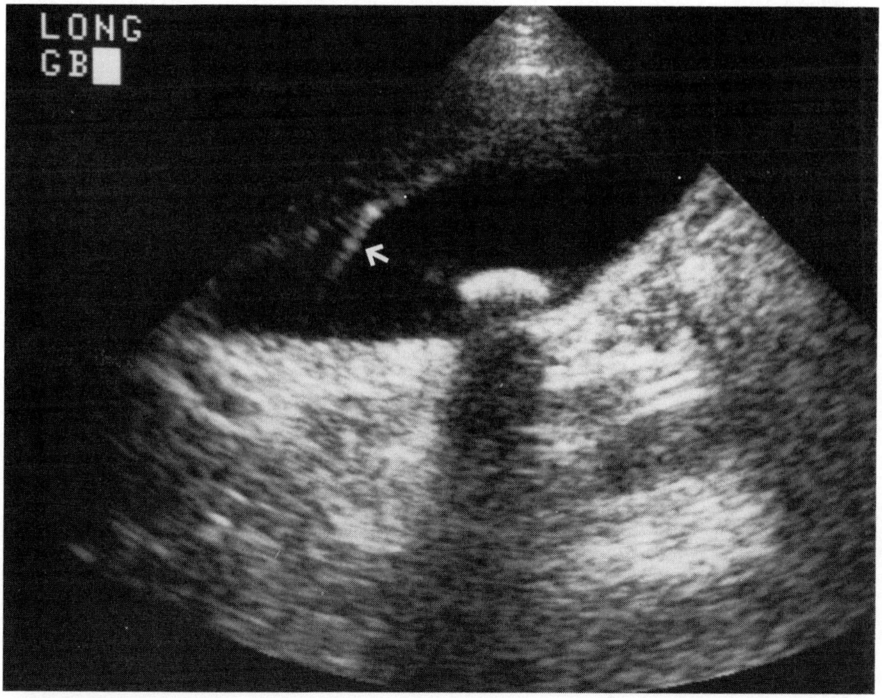

FIGURE 6. Comet-tail artifact, probably originating from the anterior gallbladder (arrow). Gallstone with "dirty" acoustic shadow is also present.

Modifying beam angulation and repositioning the patient can help overcome this often confusing artifact.

Imaging the gallbladder with an ultrasound transducer of finite beam width can cause partial volume or slice thickness artifact. This can produce an appearance similar to that of the side-lobe artifact,[7] and is minimized by utilizing a narrower sound beam and scanning through the middle of the viscus.

Several other ultrasound artifacts commonly encountered in gallbladder imaging include the ring-down artifact, the comet-tail artifact, and the V-shaped artifact. The ring-down artifact produces an echogenic band or series of bands that radiate from air-containing structures. This artifact originates from a small fluid collection trapped within a cluster of four bubbles called a bubble tetrahedron.[8] When struck by the insonating sound beam, this small fluid collection resonates, emitting a continuous soundwave that is directed back toward the transducer, producing multiple periodic bands of increased echogenicity.

The comet-tail artifact produces a series of parallel echogenic bands (Figure 6) radiating from a source which, as its name implies, resembles a comet tail. Though its sonographic appearance resembles the ring-down

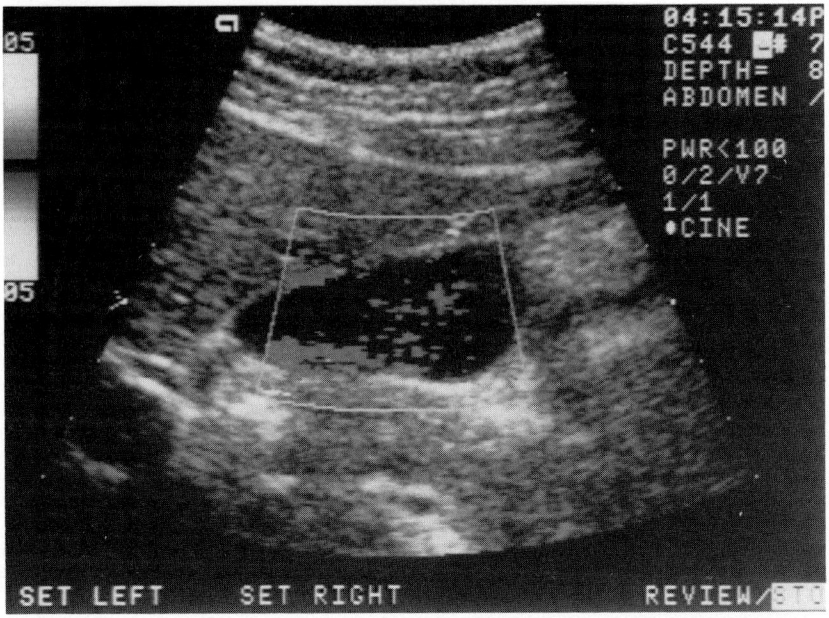

FIGURE 7. The gray areas within the box represent color flash artifact on color Doppler imaging.

artifact, its origin is different. The comet-tail artifact is caused by reverberation of the ultrasound beam within an artifact source, usually a foreign body.[9] Although it is most commonly associated with metallic foreign bodies, it can originate from other structures, such as small cholesterol crystals in postlithotripsy patients.[10]

The V-shaped artifact[11] consists of a short, V-shaped focus of increased echogenicity often seen in the anterior wall of the gallbladder. It is smaller than the comet-tail artifact and originates from small intramural cholesterol stones. This artifact results from either a strong acoustic mismatch of the stone to the insonating beam or from reverberation within the cholesterol crystals of the stone.

When performing Doppler examination in the upper abdomen, any of the typical Doppler artifacts may be seen. A color flash artifact of the gallbladder has been described and is caused by transducer motion, which preferentially places a flash of color in the normally anechoic gallbladder lumen.[12] This artifact is prevented by holding the transducer still and minimizing any patient motion (Figure 7).

Computed tomography is generally not utilized to specifically study the gallbladder. However, its wide field of view is useful in evaluating patients with nonspecific abdominal pain and in assessing abdominal pain in the obese patient, an area in which ultrasound evaluation can be limited.

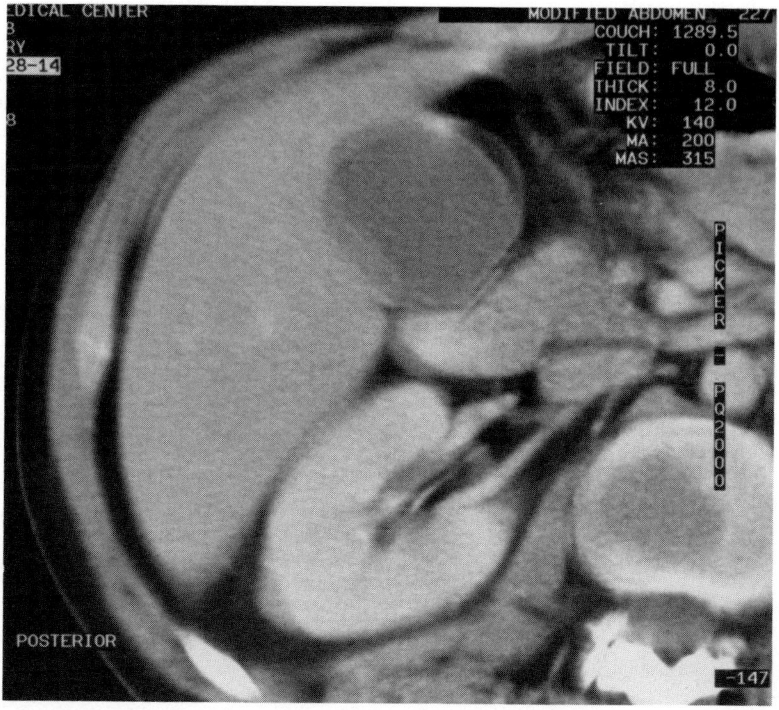

FIGURE 8. Extensive breathing artifact is seen involving the gallbladder and surrounding structures, which can mimic pericholecystic fluid.

Several artifacts are frequently encountered in CT and should be readily recognized. Patient motion (usually breathing motion) is common in acutely ill patients and can mimic the presence of pericholecystic fluid, gallbladder wall thickening, or sludge (Figure 8). Partial volume artifacts can also mimic pathology such as gallstones or intraluminal masses (Figure 16, Chapter 9). Attention to detail and re-imaging the areas in question allows such artifacts to be more readily recognized, preventing misdiagnosis.

Although the clinical utility of MRI in assessing gallbladder disease has yet to be defined, the reader should recognize several frequently occurring imaging artifacts. Aliasing or wrap-around artifacts, relatively common in MRI, occur when a portion of the patient extends beyond the field of view. Due to image sampling, a portion of the patient anatomy appears to wrap around the image, overlapping the opposite side.[13] These artifacts can occur in the frequency-encoding, phase-encoding, or slice-encoding directions. Although techniques for oversampling reduce their incidence, occasionally these artifacts can mimic disease.

Ghosting artifacts, the most prevalent of all MRI artifacts, are faint duplications of all or part of an image. Periodic patient motion (from breathing, bowel peristalsis, or vascular pulsation) in the phase-encoding direction[13] is the most common source of ghosting. Although the repetitive nature of these artifacts readily distinguishes them as ghosts, they can occasionally mimic abnormality.

REFERENCES

1. **Kremkau, F. W., Ed.,** *Diagnostic Ultrasound Principles, Instruments, and Exercises,* 3rd ed., W. B. Saunders, Philadelphia, 1989.
2. **Kremkau, F. W. and Taylor, K. J.,** Artifacts in ultrasound imaging, *J. Ultrasound Med.,* 5, 227, 1986.
3. **Thieme, G. A.,** Clinical relevance of scattering, in *Ultrasound Scattering in Biological Tissues,* Shung, K. K. and Thieme, G. A., Eds., CRC Press, Boca Raton, FL, 1993, chap. 2.
4. **Sommer, F. G., Filly, R. A., and Monton, M. J.,** Acoustic shadowing due to refractive and reflective effects, *AJR,* 132, 973, 1979.
5. **Robinson, D. E., Wilson, L. S., and Kossoff, G.,** Shadowing and enhancement in ultrasonic echograms by reflection and refraction, *J. Clin. Ultrasound,* 9, 181, 1981.
6. **Laing, F. C. and Kurtz, A. B.,** The importance of ultrasonic side-lobe artifacts, *Radiology,* 145, 763, 1982.
7. **Fiske, C. E. and Filly, R. A.,** Pseudo-sludge, *Radiology,* 144, 631, 1982.
8. **Avruch, L. and Cooperberg, P. L.,** The ring-down artifact, *J. Ultrasound Med.,* 4, 21, 1985.
9. **Ziskin, M. C., Thickman, D. I., Goldenberg, N. J., Lapayowker, M. S., and Becker, J. M.,** The comet tail artifact, *J. Ultrasound Med.,* 1, 1, 1982.
10. **Shapiro, R. S. and Winsberg, F.,** Comet-tail artifact from cholesterol crystals: observations in the postlithotripsy gallbladder and an in vitro model, *Radiology,* 177, 153, 1990.
11. **Lafortune, M., Gariepy, G., Dumont, A., Breton, G., and Lapointe, R.,** The V-shaped artifact of the gallbladder wall, *AJR,* 147, 505, 1986.
12. **Pozniak, M. A., Zagzebski, J. A., and Scanlan, K. A.,** Spectral and color doppler artifacts, *Radiographics,* 12, 35, 1992.
13. **Henkelman, R. M.,** Image artifacts, in *Magnetic Resonance Imaging,* 2nd ed., Stark, D. D. and Bradley, W. G., Jr., Eds., Mosby Year Book, St. Louis, 1992, chap. 10.

Chapter 9

PSEUDOLESIONS

Jon W. Meilstrup, Kenneth D. Hopper, and Claudia J. Kasales

Occasionally gallbladder images mimic true pathologic conditions. An awareness of these common pseudolesions can prevent their misdiagnosis as disease. The technical artifacts that can mimic disease have been discussed previously (see Chapter 8). This chapter focuses on the appearance of the gallbladder which initially may suggest abnormality, but with closer evaluation is actually normal.[1]

Some of these pseudolesions have been mentioned in other chapters. Folds can mimic stones on sonography when the ultrasound beam is perpendicular to the fold causing posterior shadowing.[2] Gallbladder folds can also mimic actual septations.

The gallbladder can occasionally assume an unusual shape due to tortuosity or bending, such as a Z-shape or curved (''boomerang'') appearance. A ''boomerang'' gallbladder on longitudinal sonography shows a gentle curve resembling the shape of the letter ''C''; however, on transverse sonography and computed tomography (CT), the gallbladder appears as two separate cystic structures. Without the parasagittal view, one of these cystic areas may be mistaken to represent a pseudocyst[3] (Figure 1), cystic mass, or even gallbladder duplication[4] (Figure 2).

One common source of gallbladder pseudolesions is related to camera recording of images. On older cameras with mirror technology, so-called moon spots appeared on some images, not only overlying the gallbladder, but other structures and the image background as well (Figure 3). This pseudolesion results from dust on the imaging mirror of the camera, and if seen overlying the gallbladder, can mimic a mass.[5] Newer digital recording devices have overcome such distractions, but electronic artifacts still may be seen.

Varying appearances of the bile in the gallbladder have been noted. On sonography, low-level echoes can occur as the result of increased cholesterol crystal content (Figure 4), although other causes are possible.[6–10] Thick bile, or sludge (Figure 5), is also readily seen on sonography with a reported prevalence up to 0.21%.[8] It is seen in fasting patients, as well as those on hyperalimentation, and can be found in patients with cholestasis, nonbiliary sepsis, and pancreatitis.[5,10] Sometimes echogenic bile fills the gallbladder, making it appear similar to the echogenicity of adjacent liver. This echogenic, sludge-filled appearance is called sonographic ''hepatization'' of the gallbladder[4,11] (Figure 6).

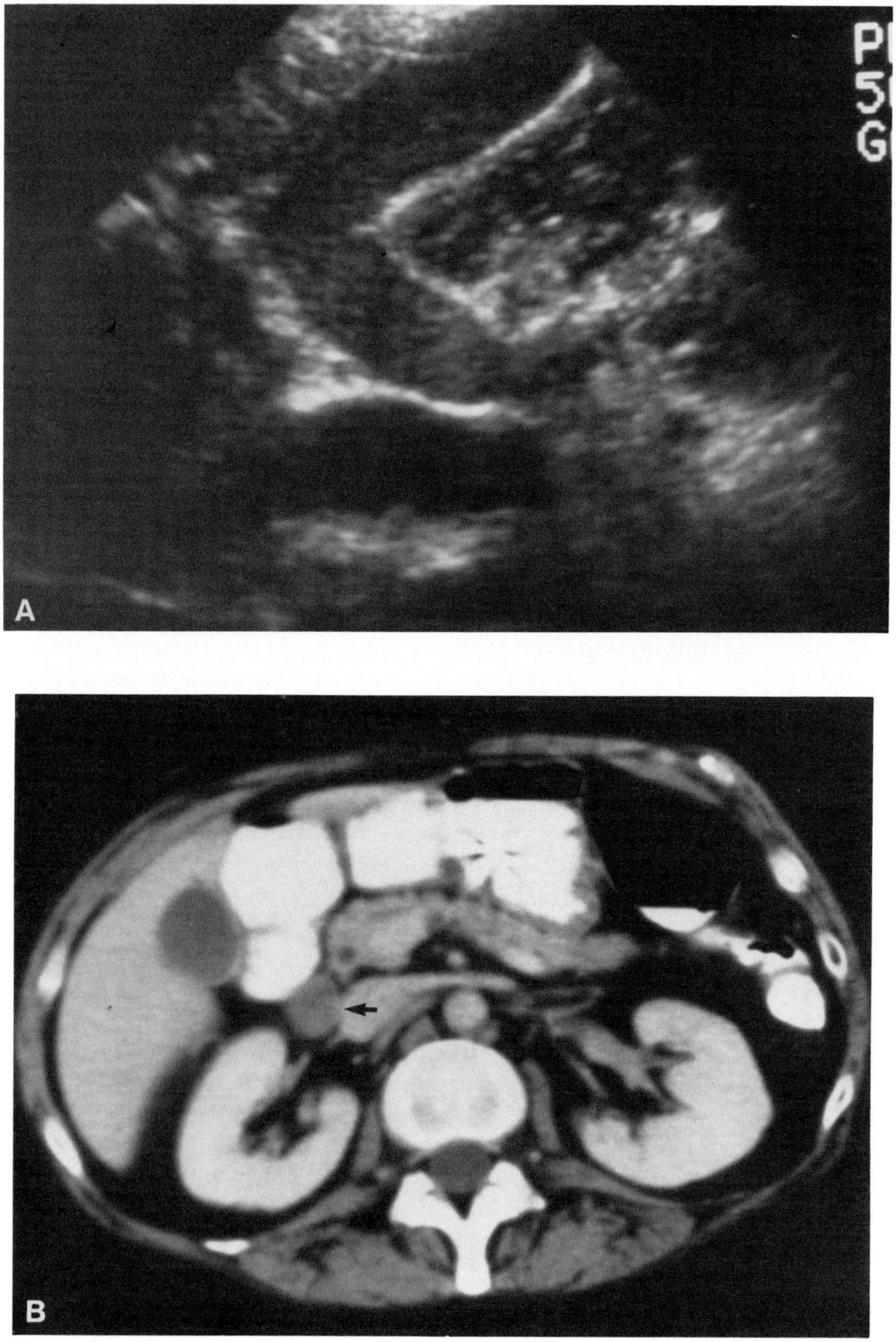

FIGURE 1. (A) Tight curve in a sludge-filled gallbladder produces a ''boomerang'' shape on longitudinal sonogram; CT section (B) through this gallbladder mimics a pseudocyst near the head of the pancreas (arrow). (From Meilstrup, J. W., Hopper, K. D., and Thieme, G. A., *AJR,* 157, 1205, 1991. With permission.)

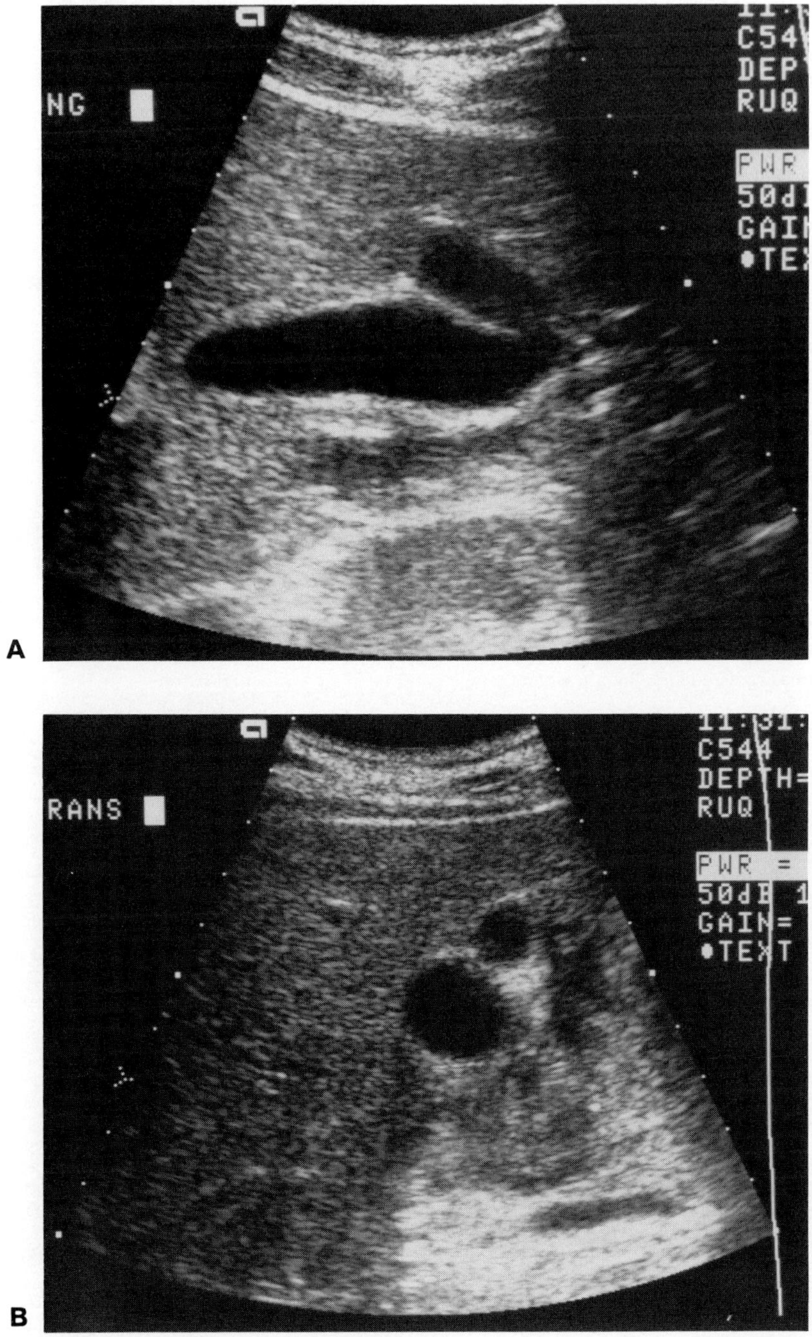

FIGURE 2. Very tight curve in this gallbladder on a longitudinal sonography (A) mimics gallbladder duplication on the transverse view (B).

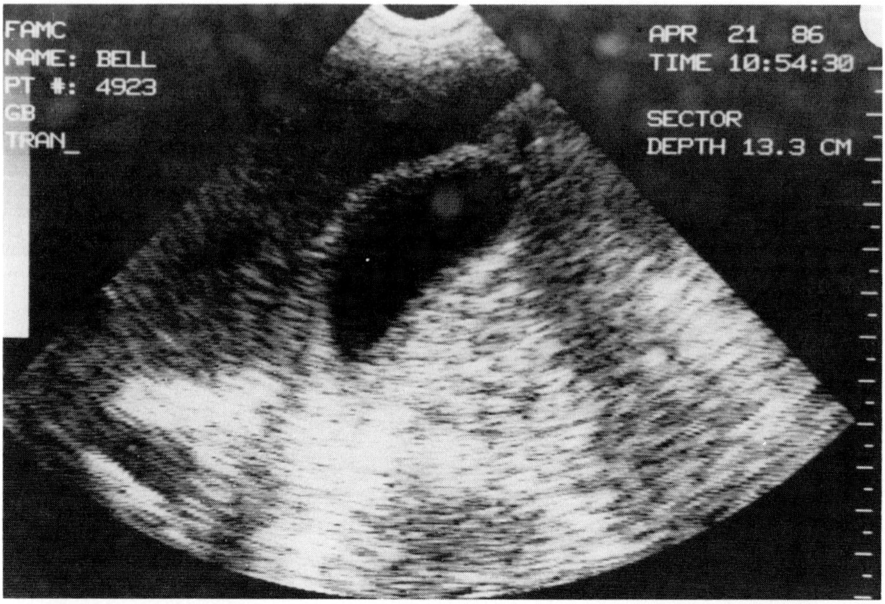

FIGURE 3. Dust particles (''moon spots'') on the camera mirror can produce pseudolesions, which might be confusing if they overlie the gallbladder, as in this case, but the presence of similar spots outside the ultrasound image confirms their artifactual nature.

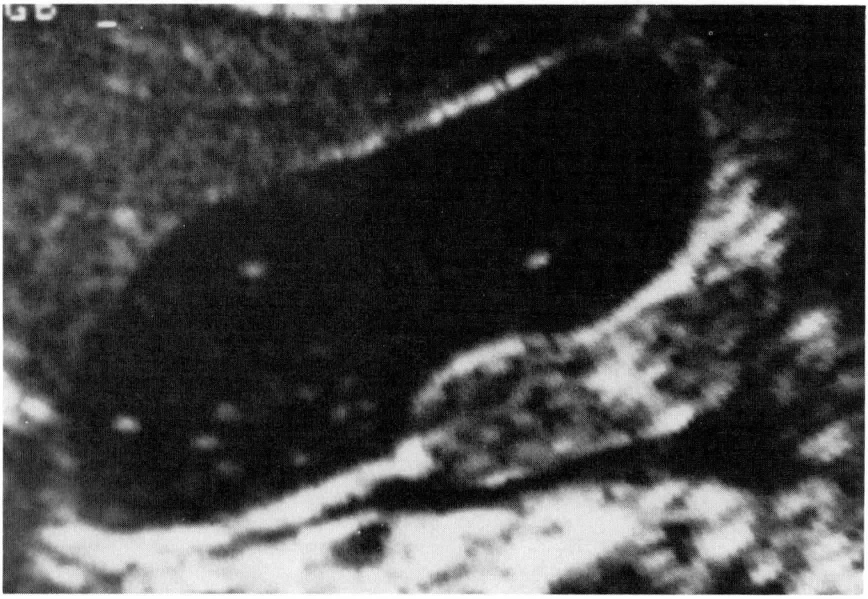

FIGURE 4. Diffuse low-level echoes can be noted in bile due to increased content of cholesterol crystals.

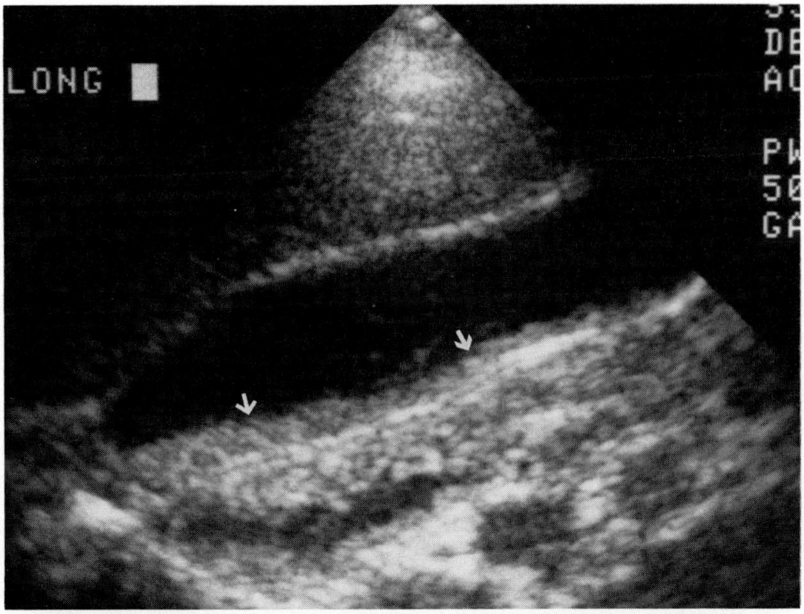

A

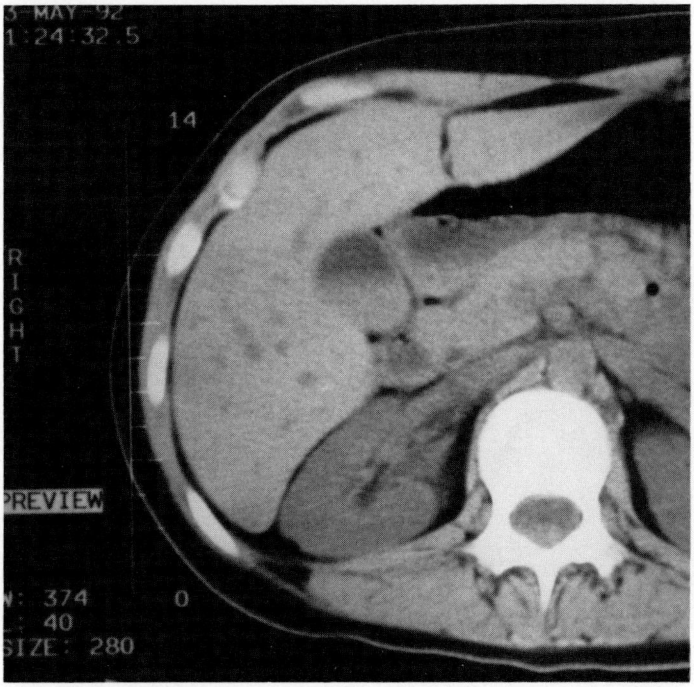

B

FIGURE 5. Sludge or thick bile can layer (arrows), and appears more echogenic on sonography (A) or more dense on CT (B) than does normal bile.

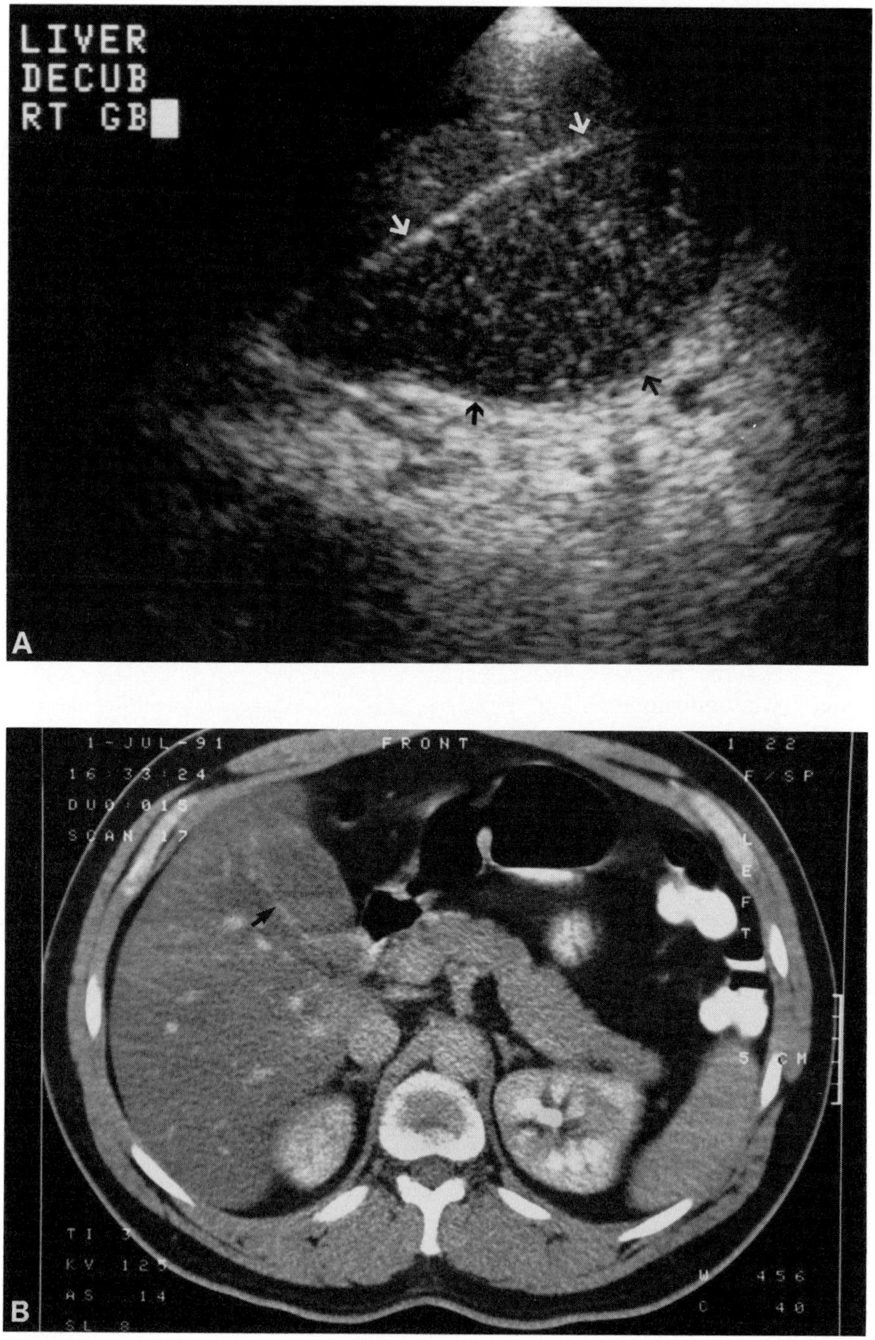

FIGURE 6. Sludge may fill the gallbladder (arrows), and appear similar to the liver, (''hepatization'' of the gallbladder). (A) Longitudinal sonogram, (B) contrast-enhanced CT.

The two major components of sludge are calcium bilirubinate and cholesterol crystals,[12] both in a matrix of mucus gel.[13] The appearance of sludge is variable and related to its viscosity and composition. However, sludge generally layers in the dependent position, with less dense bile more anterior. Occasionally sludge can appear as a viscous mass, referred to as ''tumefactive sludge'',[14,15] which typically changes shape very slowly with different patient positions (Figure 7). Because focal gallbladder sludge typically has a ''soft echogenic pattern'' and no acoustic shadow, it may be difficult to differentiate from a mass. Repeat examinations may be necessary to demonstrate change in its position or shape.[14] A relationship of sludge to the formation of stones has been postulated, but is still unproven. Sludge has rarely formed ball-like masses resembling stones.[6] Milk-of-calcium bile may resemble sludge but is usually more echogenic[5,16] or radiodense (Figure 8; Chapter 5, Figure 5B).

On normal sonography, CT, magnetic resonance imaging (MRI), and oral cholecystography, a layering of bile of differing specific gravity is sometimes seen.[17] This appears as layers of differing echogenicity on sonography, different densities on CT, and different signal intensities on MRI (Figure 5, Chapter 2). When a patient is supine, this layering of bile may produce an ''edge-ring effect'' on contrast studies, which can simulate a large gallstone; however, after adequate mixing of the contrast medium and bile, this pseudostone will not be seen.

Composed mostly of water, normal bile is iso-osmotic to plasma. Its density on CT, therefore, is similar to that of a simple cyst. The administration of intravenous contrast does not acutely affect the attenuation of bile. While the gallbladder wall normally enhances after the administration of i.v. contrast,[18] the excretion of contrast into bile is less frequently encountered. This ''vicarious excretion'' has been noted in patients with renal failure,[19] and acute unilateral ureteral obstruction,[20] but it may also occur in normal patients, especially when higher doses of contrast medium are used.[21–23] The dense gallbladder from vicarious excretion may persist for several hours (Figure 9). Correlation with any history of recent radiologic studies is necessary to differentiate vicarious excretion of contrast from other entities such as milk-of-calcium bile.

The clinical utility of MRI in the assessment of gallbladder disease is not yet established. The appearance of bile on MRI is variable, and depends upon the relative concentration of water and lipids.[24] Bile recently produced by the liver contains a large amount of water. As a result, its signal intensity follows that of water on spin echo sequences. Bile that has been present within the gallbladder for several hours, however, is concentrated and has a higher lipid content, shortening its T1 value as compared to recently produced bile (Figure 5A, Chapter 2).

After biliary and gastric surgery, oral contrast material may enter the gallbladder, and air-contrast levels may be seen (Figure 10). At oral

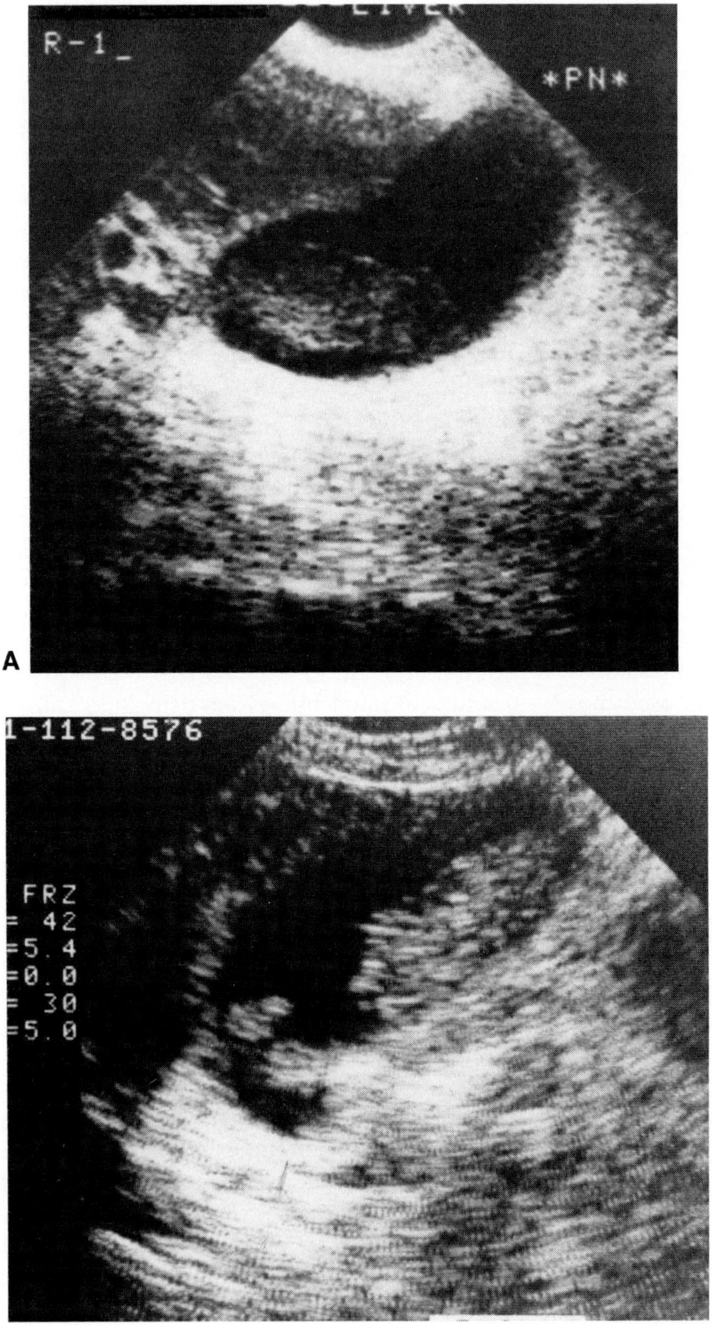

A

B

FIGURE 7. (A, B) Tumefactive sludge in two different patients.

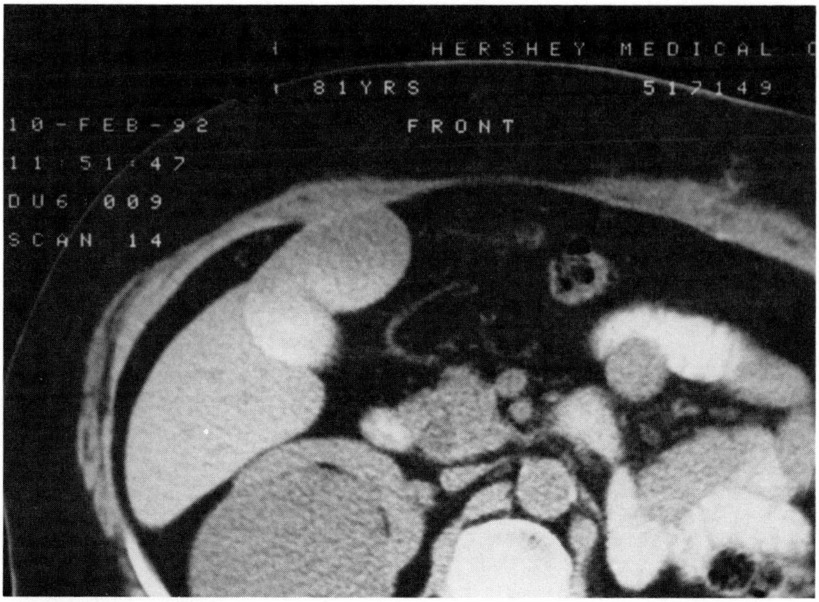

FIGURE 8. Milk of calcium bile appears as increased attenuation in the gallbladder, as on this unenhanced CT image.

cholecystography, contrast medium may precipitate in the gallbladder lumen, and can simulate gallstones.[17] Sonography can demonstrate echogenic foci within the gallbladder from food particles entering after cholecystojejunostomy.[25]

The normal gallbladder wall is thin, and is especially well seen on sonography and enhanced CT. Gallbladder wall thickening ($\geq$3 mm) is a nonspecific sign and may be normal if the gallbladder is contracted (Figure 11). However, many pathologic entities have been described which cause gallbladder wall thickening,[5,26] including cholecystitis (acute and chronic), hypoalbuminemia, hepatitis, acquired immunodeficiency syndrome, congestive heart failure, portal adenopathy, infiltrative gallbladder masses, adenomyomatosis, and neoplasm. Pseudothickening of the gallbladder wall is seen with ascites and with breathing artifact on CT and MRI (Figure 12).

One pseudolesion unique to CT occurs when the gallbladder wall is thickened and edematous.[27] The wall may appear poorly defined and of decreased attenuation, mimicking fluid or bile. The enhancing gallbladder mucosa, displaced centrally by the edematous wall, gives the appearance of a rounded focus of increased attenuation, which resembles a stone within a small, bile-filled gallbladder. The relative position of this pseudostone (central location as opposed to a true dependent position) and its relatively increased length (gallstones are generally round or oval) are clues aiding differentiation of this artifact from true stones.

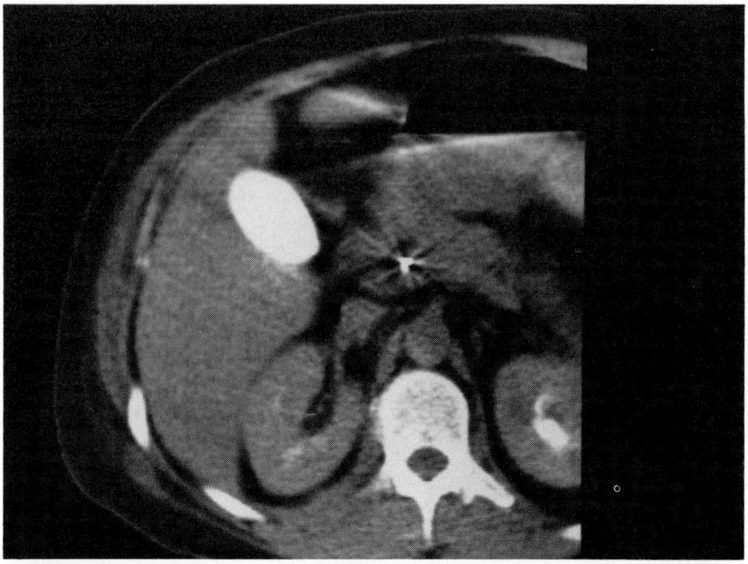

A

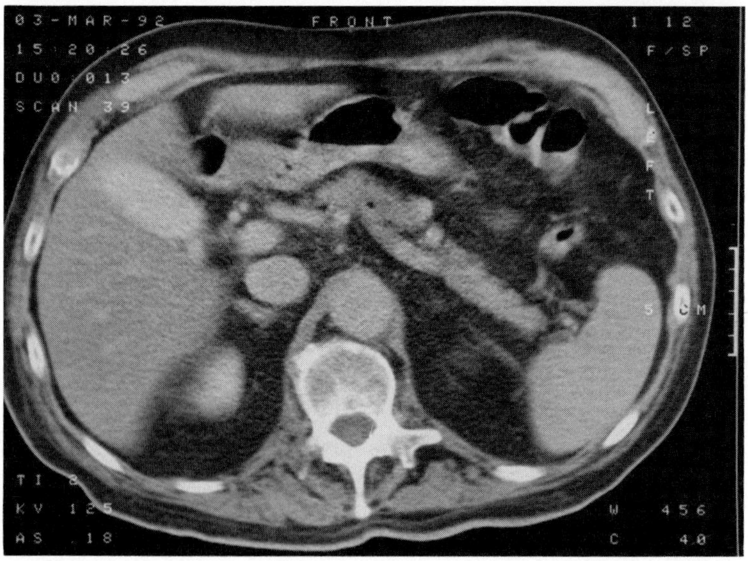

B

FIGURE 9. Vicarious excretion. The gallbladder shows high attenuation values on the CT images of a patient (A) who had acute ureteral obstruction; the gallbladder displays ''vicarious excretion'' of i.v. contrast medium. While this is seen in patients with renal failure or urinary obstruction, it may also be seen in patients with normal renal function, as in this 86-year-old male (B). Occasionally, vicarious excretion can also be seen with other water-soluble contrast media, such as intrathecal, intraarterial, and endoscopic retrograde cholecystic pancreatography agents, as well as with oral water-soluble media.

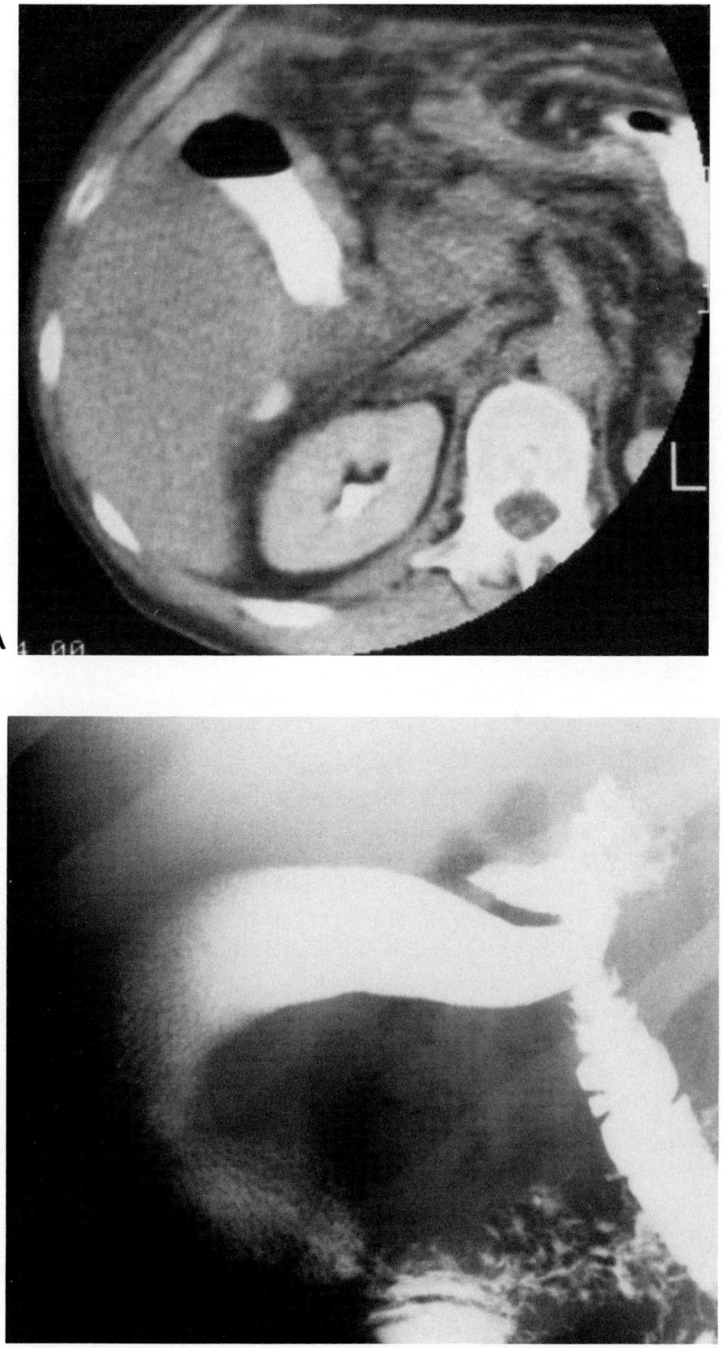

A

B

FIGURE 10. Reflux opacification of the gallbladder (A) with gastrografin is seen as an air-contrast level on this CT section, secondary to a choledochojejunostomy, and (B) with barium, the gallbladder showing a ''barium on velvet'' appearance after an upper GI series.

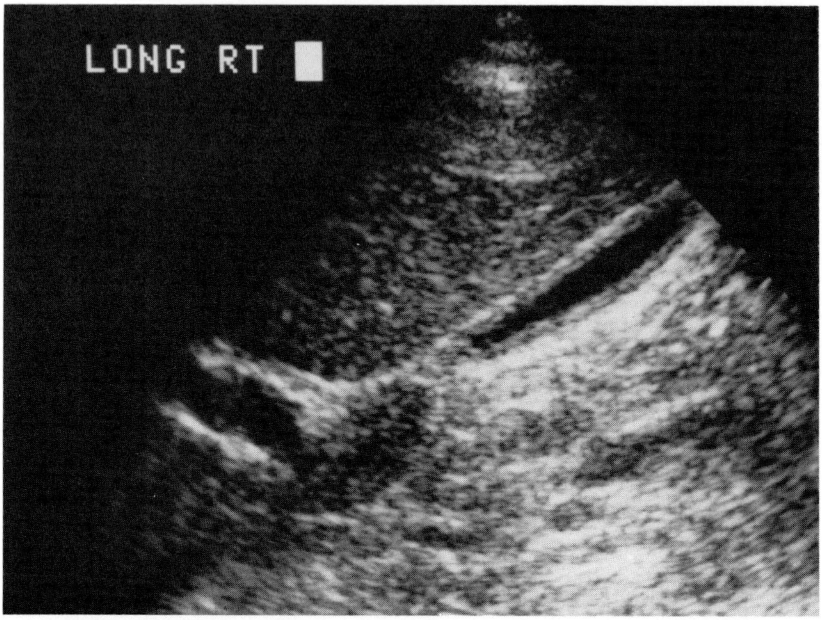

FIGURE 11. A normal contracted gallbladder on sonography will show wall thickening; this resolves after adequate fasting and gallbladder distension.

Pseudomasses of the gallbladder are common. On sonography, the duodenum is generally easily recognized by its air-filled lumen, location, and typical appearance. Occasionally, however, the duodenum mimics a mass or stone (Figure 13). On sonography or CT, the fluid-filled duodenum can also appear as a pseudo-gallbladder[28] (Figure 14). A dilated afferent loop in a patient with afferent loop syndrome has been reported to cause a similar appearance.[29] Fluid in the duodenum can also mimic gallbladder duplication on plain film radiographs.[17] Real-time ultrasound scanning usually resolves these pseudolesions. However, if any question remains, the patient can be given water orally, and duodenal peristalsis readily identified.

Sometimes the duodenum can mimic the gallbladder on scintigraphy.[30] Bile leakage into the gallbladder fossa has also mimicked a gallbladder on hepatobiliary scintigraphy.[31] The gallbladder also can be visualized when using nonbiliary radiopharmaceuticals, for example, ^{99m}Tc bone scans and red blood cell imaging.[32,33]

Sonography in certain planes can produce pseudomasses in the gallbladder (Figure 15), which are clarified on perpendicular views; transverse CT images can also produce these pseudolesions (Figure 16). Careful scanning and comparison with the image above and below the section in question will provide the answer. Occasionally, a pseudomass may be seen on radiographic studies when a Phrygian cap or the gallbladder neck is seen *en face.* If, however, a luminal mass remains constant on multiple sonographic or CT sections, the possibility of a gallbladder mass, polyp, or even heterotopic gastric mucosa must be considered.[34]

A

B

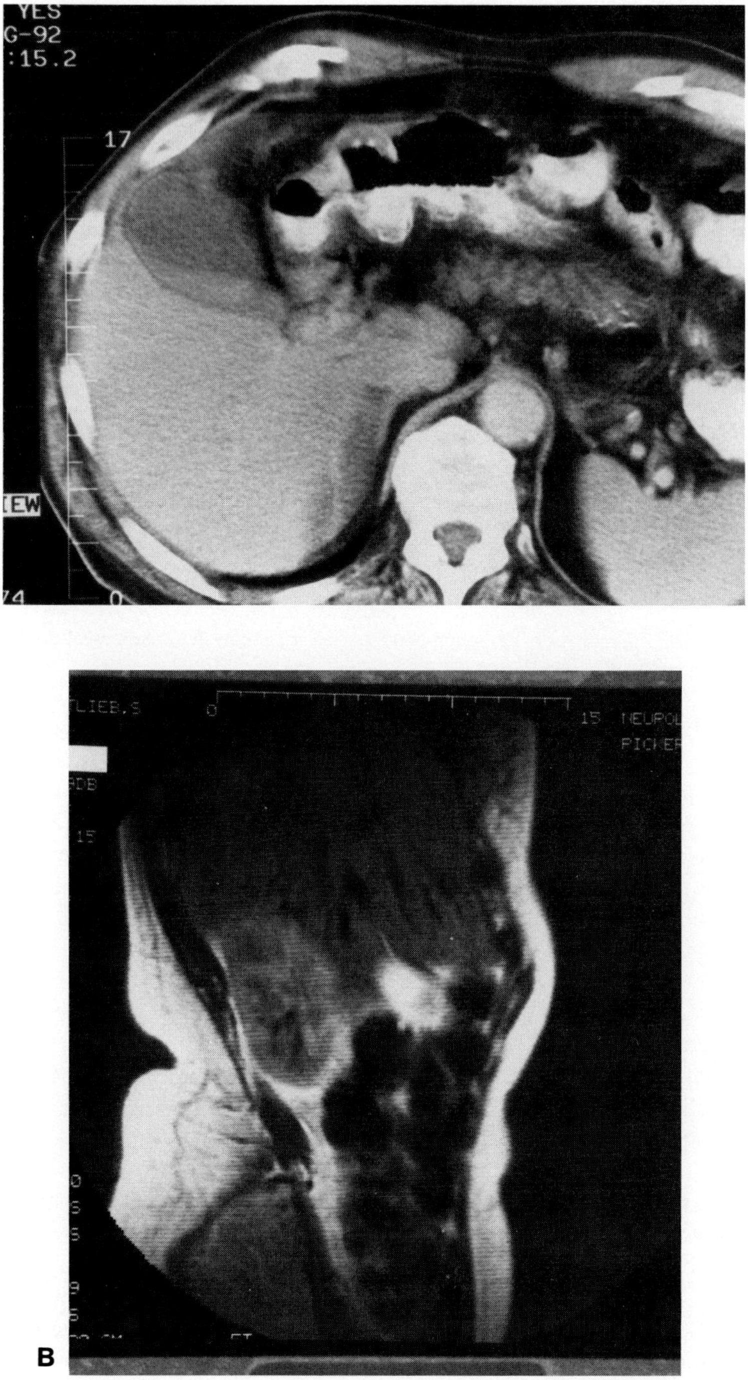

FIGURE 12. With patient breathing artifact, the gallbladder wall can appear spuriously thickened, as on this CT section (A). Breathing or motion artifact (such as bowel peristalsis) can mimic sludge, or can even mimic an intraluminal mass, as on this parasagittal T1-weighted MRI (B).

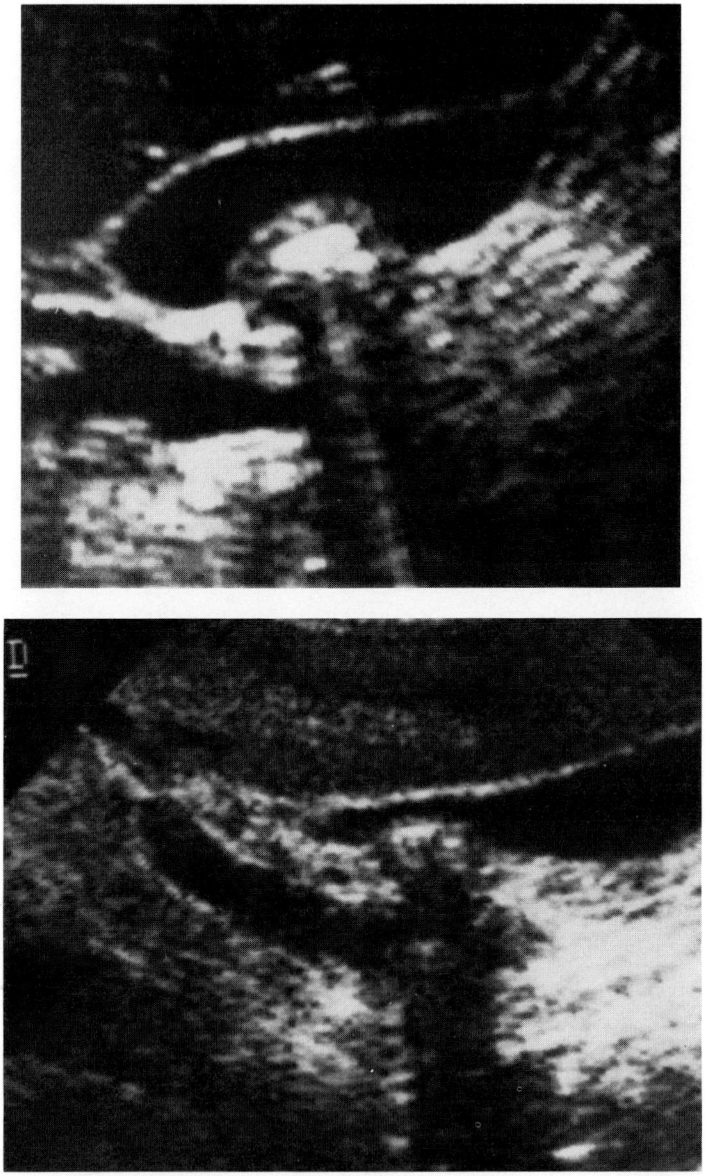

A

B

FIGURE 13. The duodenum can mimic gallbladder masses on sonography. Usually an echogenic center emanates from the air and/or mucus in the duodenum (A), and the duodenum will show peristalsis over the examination time. The duodenum in another patient mimics a stone with shadowing on the sonogram (B), but with peristalsis the area changes (C). Air in bowel can also mimic large stones on sonography as in this patient (D), who on further evaluation had a normal gallbladder (E). Note the marked normal folding of this C-shaped gallbladder in E.

C

D

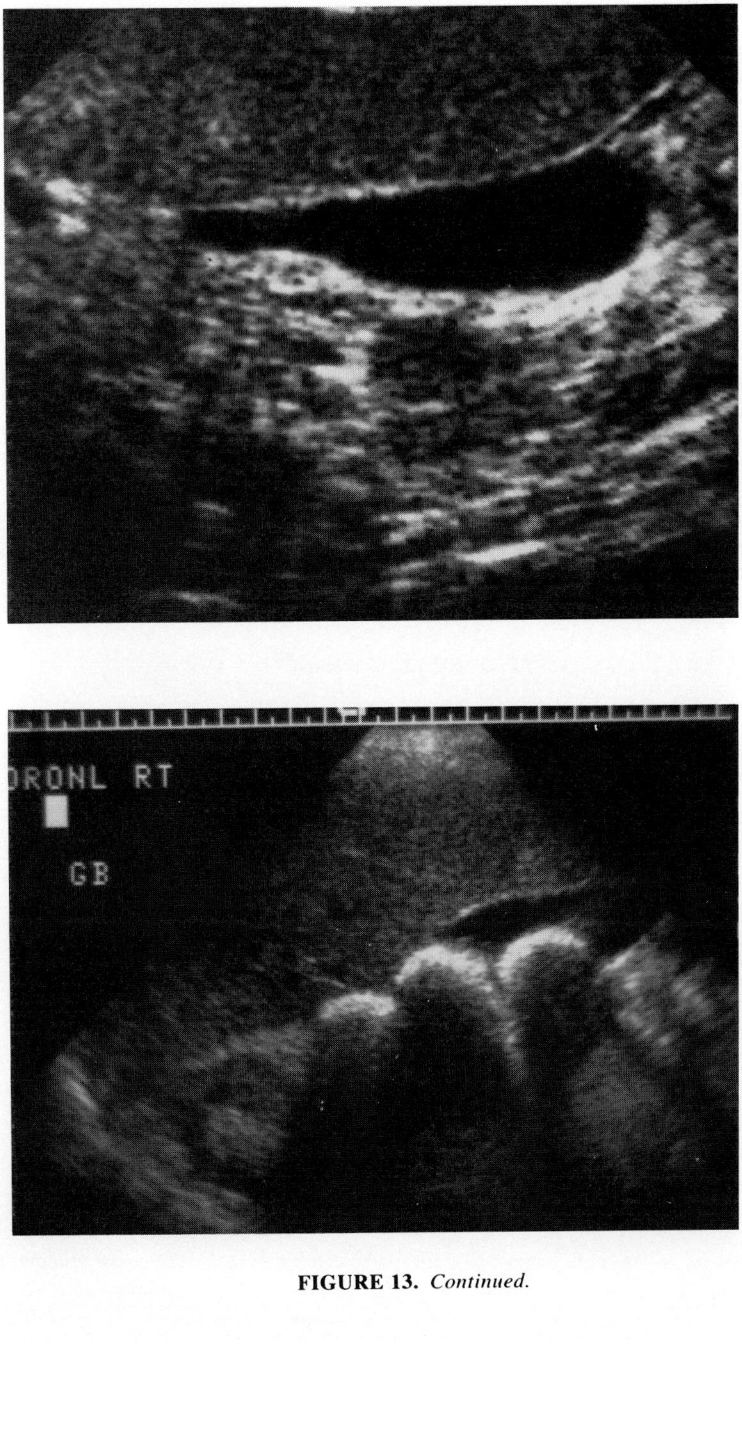

FIGURE 13. *Continued.*

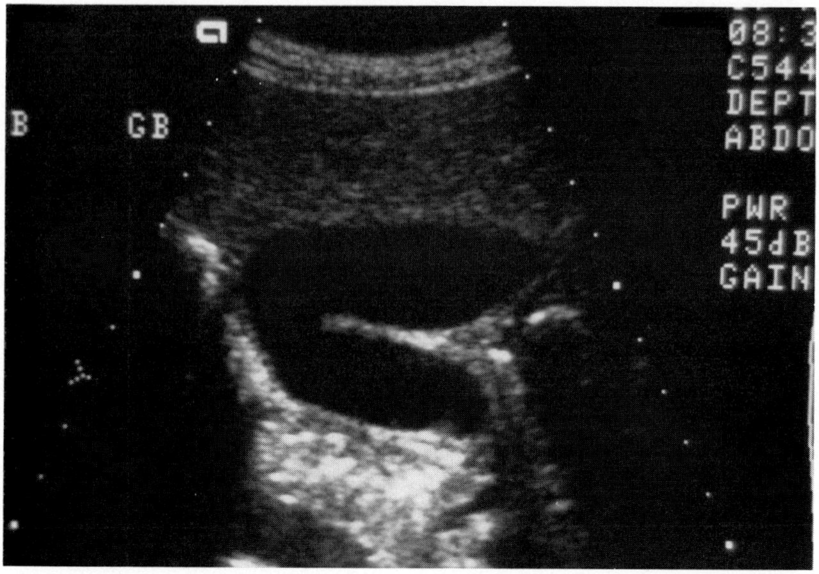

E

FIGURE 13. *Continued.*

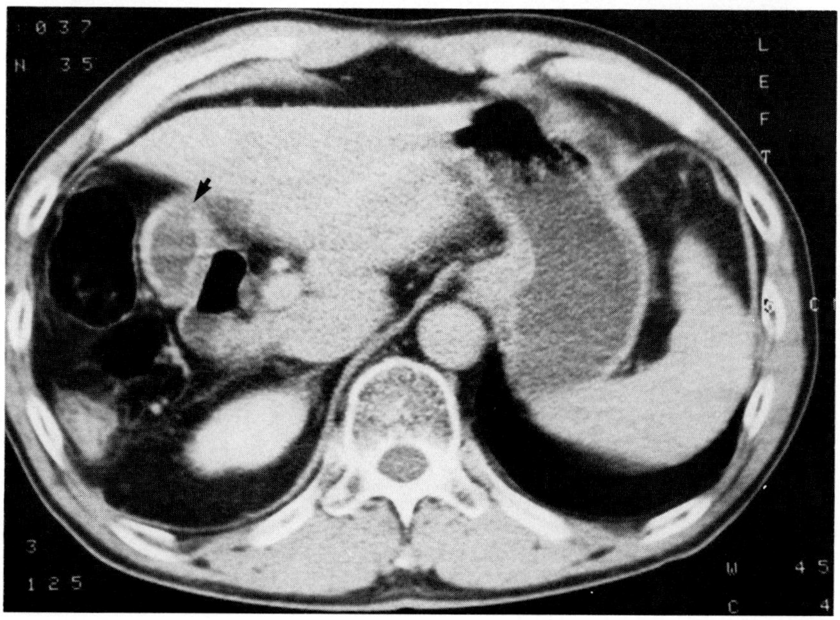

A

FIGURE 14. A fluid-filled duodenum (arrow) can mimic a gallbladder with a thickened wall on CT sections, as in this patient (A, B). Right hepatic lobe is hypoplastic. (C) An intrahepatic gallbladder (open arrow) was located cephalad to image (A).

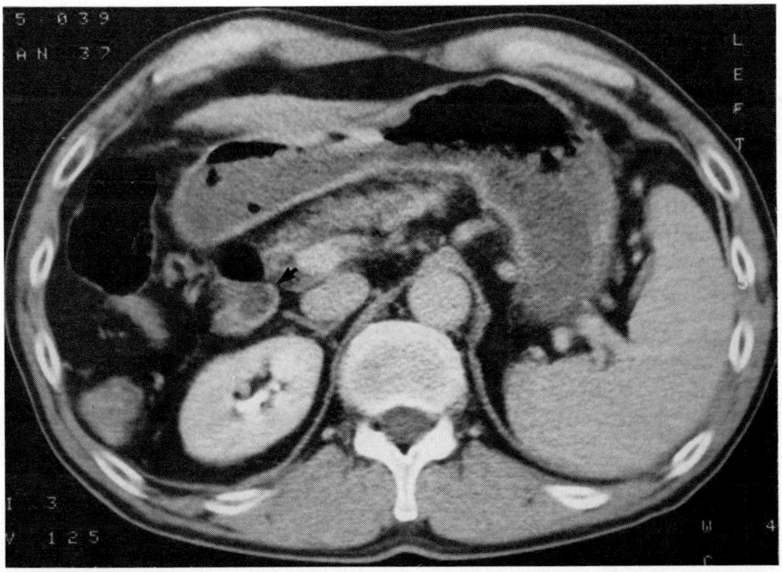

B

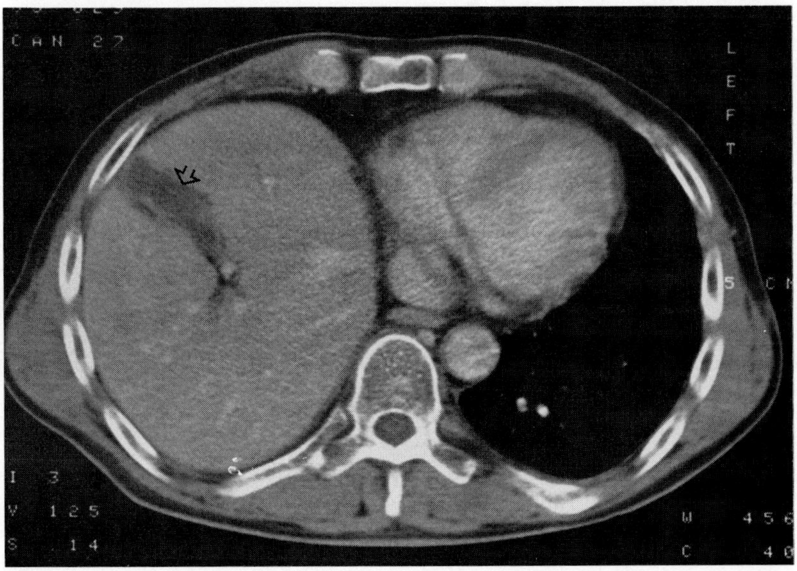

C

FIGURE 14. *Continued.*

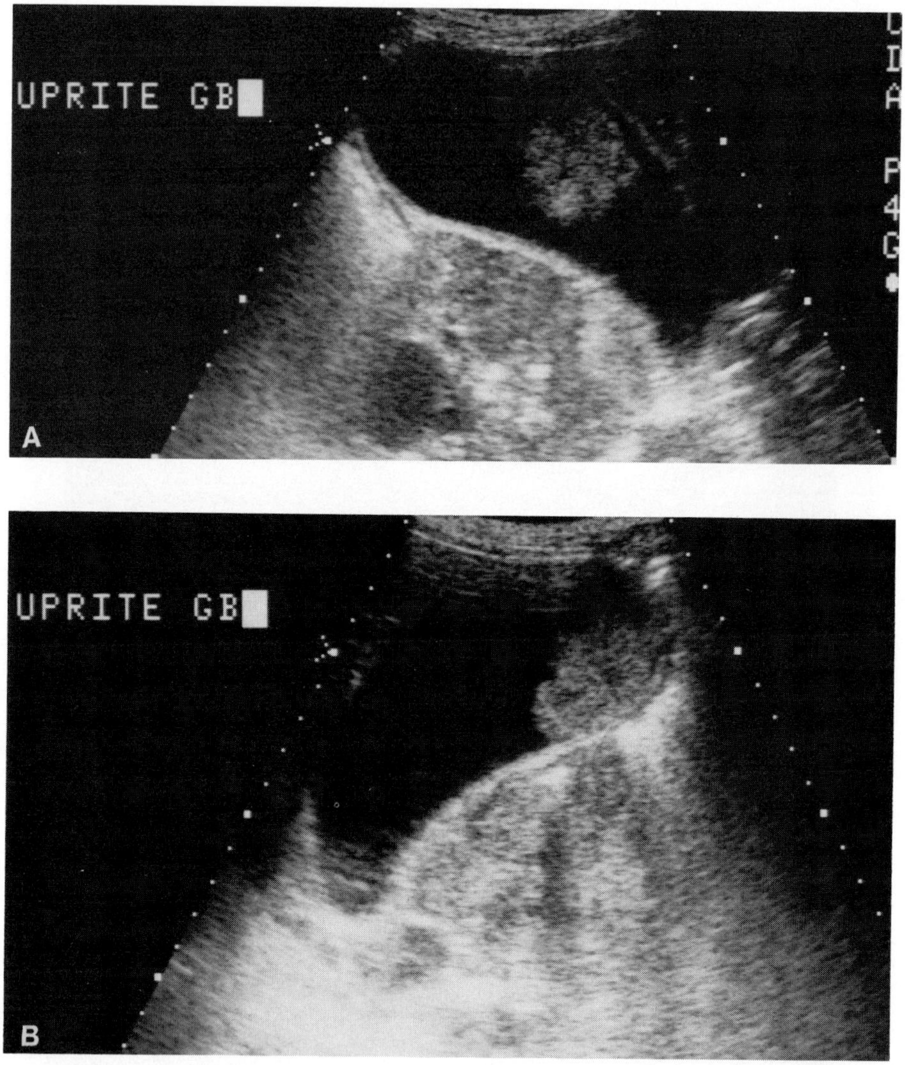

FIGURE 15. An intraluminal mass is mimicked on one sonographic view (A), but on another view (B) at right angles to (A), focal intraluminal sludge is seen to be the source of the pseudomass.

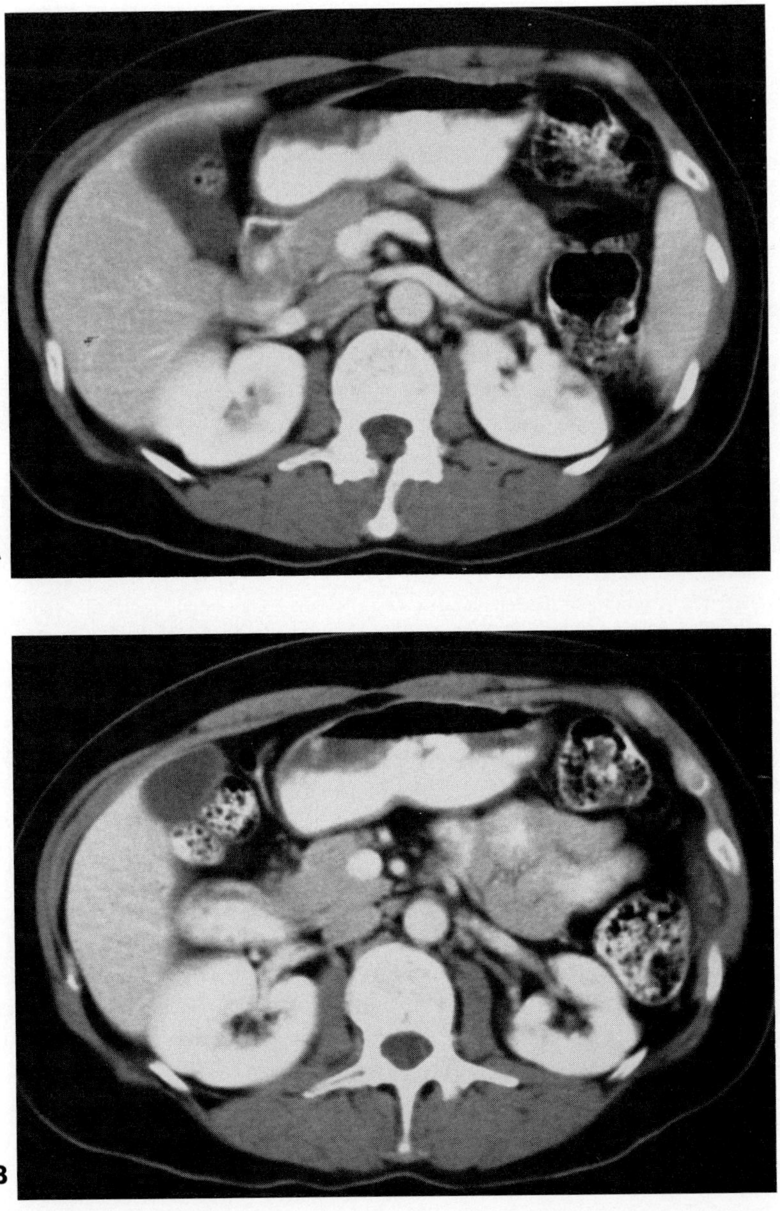

A

B

FIGURE 16. Because of volume averaging on CT, adjacent bowel can mimic an intraluminal gallbladder mass (A), which is readily recognized on the next lower section (B).

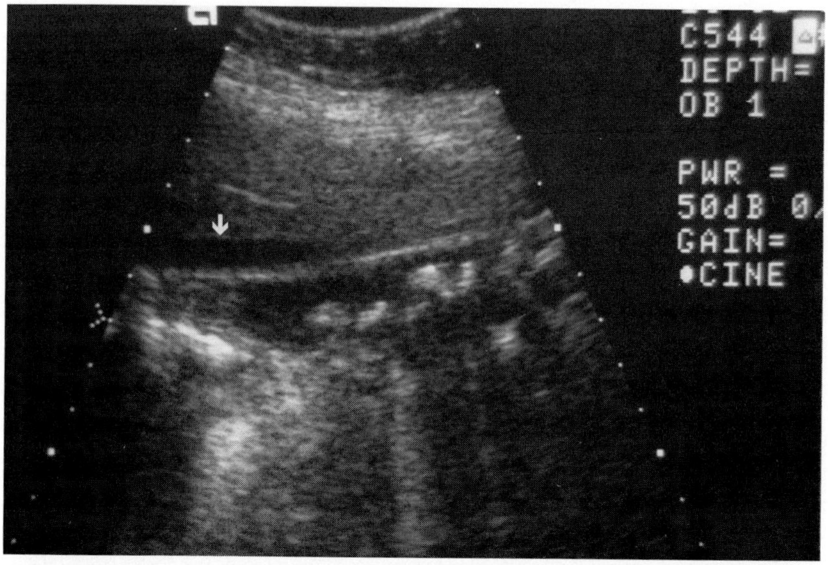

FIGURE 17. A prominent pericholecystic vessel (arrow) may mimic pericholecystic fluid; color Doppler imaging (not shown) revealed the true vascular nature of the finding. Multiple gallstones are noted.

A pericholecystic vessel or hypoechoic pericholecystic fat will rarely mimic pericholecystic fluid. Color Doppler ultrasound imaging will establish any vascular structure as a normal variant (Figure 17), while CT may be necessary to establish the low density of pericholecystic fat. Gallbladder wall varices can also mimic gallbladder wall thickening,[35] but their true nature should be obvious with Doppler examination.

As noted above, these pseudolesions are seen with virtually all imaging modalities. However, a knowledge of normal gallbladder anatomy and its broad range of variable appearances, together with careful analysis of all images, will generally allow differentiation of any pseudolesion from a real one. In the rare instance where this determination remains equivocal, a complementary imaging procedure is usually diagnostic.

REFERENCES

1. **Fitzgerald, E. J. and Toi, A.,** Pitfalls in the ultrasonographic diagnosis of gallbladder diseases, *Postgrad. Med. J.*, 63, 525, 1987.
2. **Sukov, R. J., Sample, F., Sarti, D. A., and Whitcomb, M. J.,** Cholecystosonography—the junctional fold, *Radiology*, 133, 435, 1979.
3. **Meilstrup, J. W., Hopper, K. D., and Thieme, G. A.,** Imaging of gallbladder variants, *AJR*, 157, 1205, 1991.
4. **Hammond, D. I.,** Unusual causes of sonographic nonvisualization or nonrecognition of the gallbladder: a review, *J. Clin. Ultrasound*, 16, 77, 1988.
5. **Rosenthal, S. J., Cox, G. G., Wetzel, L. H., and Batnitzky, S.,** Pitfalls and differential diagnosis in biliary sonography, *RadioGraphics*, 10, 285, 1990.
6. **Jeanty, P., Ammann, W., Cooperberg, P., Gooding, G. A. W., Kunstlinger, F., LeClerg, F., and van Gansbeke, D.,** Mobile intraluminal masses of the gallbladder, *J. Ultrasound Med.*, 2, 65, 1983.
7. **Glancy, J. J., Goddard, J., and Pearson, D. E.,** In vitro demonstration of cholesterol crystals' high echogenicity relative to protein particles, *J. Clin. Ultrasound*, 8, 27, 1980.
8. **Angelico, M., DeSantis, A., and Capocaccia, L.,** Biliary sludge: a critical update, *J. Clin. Gastroenterol.*, 12, 656, 1990.
9. **Simeone, J. F., Mueller, P. R., Ferucci, J. T., Jr., Harbin, W. P., and Wittenberg, J.,** Significance of nonshadowing focal opacities at cholecystosonography, *Radiology*, 137, 181, 1980.
10. **Conrad, M. R., Janes, J. O., and Dietchy, J.,** Significance of low-level echoes within the gallbladder, *AJR*, 132, 967, 1979.
11. **Reining, J. W. and Stanley, J. H.,** Sonographic hepatization of the gallbladder: a cause of nonvisualization of the gallbladder by cholecystosonography, *J. Clin. Ultrasound*, 12, 234, 1984.
12. **Filly, R. A., Allen, B., Minton, M. J., Bernhoft, R., and Way, L. W.,** In vitro investigation of the origin of echoes within biliary sludge, *J. Clin. Ultrasound*, 8, 193, 1980.
13. **Ohara, N. and Schaefer, J.,** Clinical significance of biliary sludge, *J. Clin. Gastroenterol.*, 12, 291, 1990.
14. **Fakhry, J.,** Sonography of tumefactive biliary sludge, *AJR*, 139, 717, 1982.
15. **Rahmani, M. R.,** Letter to the editor: tumefactive biliary sludge, *AJR*, 145, 860, 1985.
16. **Love, M. B.,** Sonographic features of milk of calcium bile, *J. Ultrasound Med.*, 1, 325, 1982.
17. **Keats, T. E.,** *Atlas of Normal Roentgen Variants That May Simulate Disease*, 5th ed., Mosby Year Book, St. Louis, 1992, 902.
18. **Strax, R., Toombs, B. D., Kam, J., Rauschkolb, E. N., Patel, S., and Sandler, C. M.,** Gallbladder enhancement following angiography: a normal CT finding, *J. Comput. Assist. Tomogr.*, 6, 766, 1982.
19. **Becker, J. A., Gregoire, A., Berdon, W., and Schwartz, D.,** Vicarious excretion of urographic media, *Radiology*, 90, 243, 1968.
20. **Dyer, R. B., Gilpin, J. W., Zagoria, R. J., Chen, M. Y. M., and Case, L. D.,** Vicarious contrast material excretion in patients with acute unilateral ureteral obstruction, *Radiology*, 177, 739, 1990.
21. **Shea, T. E. and Pfister, R. C.,** Opacification of the gallbladder by urographic contrast media. Reflection of an alternate excretory pathway, *AJR*, 107, 763, 1969.
22. **Lautin, E. M. and Friedman, A. C.,** Vicarious excretion of contrast media, *JAMA*, 247, 1608, 1982.

23. **Ueda, J., Hara, K., Ohishi, H., and Uchida, H.,** High density bile in the gallbladder observed by computed tomography, *J. Comput. Assist. Tomogr.*, 7, 801, 1983.
24. **Hricak, H., Filly, R. A., Margulis, A. R., Moon, K. L., Crooks, L. E., and Kaufman, L.,** Work in progress: nuclear magnetic resonance imaging of the gallbladder, *Radiology*, 147, 481, 1983.
25. **Gooding, G. A.,** Food particles in the gallbladder mimic cholelithiasis in a patient with a cholecystojejunostomy, *J. Clin. Ultrasound*, 9, 346, 1981.
26. **Ralls, P. W., Quinn, M. F., Juttner, H. U., Halls, J. M., and Boswell, W. D.,** Gallbladder wall thickening: patients without intrinsic gallbladder disease, *AJR*, 137, 65, 1981.
27. **Middleton, W. D., Thorsen, M. K., Lawson, T. L., and Foley, W. D.,** False-positive CT diagnosis of gallstones due to thickening of the gallbladder wall, *AJR*, 149, 941, 1987.
28. **Sanders, R. C.,** *Atlas of Ultrasonographic Artifacts and Variants*, 2nd ed., Mosby Year Book, St. Louis, 1992, 161.
29. **Morse, J. M. D., Lakshman, S., and Thomas, E.,** "Pseudogallbladder" appearance in partial afferent loop obstruction in a patient with cholecystectomy, *South. Med. J.*, 79, 1030, 1986.
30. **Shaffer, P. B. and Olsen, J. O.,** Differentiation of the gallbladder from the duodenum on cholescintigrams by dynamic display, *Radiology*, 145, 217, 1982.
31. **Shih, W., Duff, D., and Mostowycz, L.,** Bile leakage accumulating in the gallbladder bed mimicking normal visualization of gallbladder in technetium-99m Disida hepatobiliary imaging, *Clin. Nucl. Med.*, 14, 222, 1989.
32. **Sherkow, L., Ryo, U. Y., Fabich, D., Patel, G. C., and Pinsky, S. M.,** Visualization of the liver, gallbladder, and intestine on bone scintigraphy, *Clin. Nucl. Med.*, 9, 440, 1984.
33. **Kotlyarov, E. V., Mattay, V. S., and Reba, R. C.,** Gallbladder visualization during technetium-99m RBC blood pool imaging, *Clin. Nucl. Med.*, 13, 515, 1988.
34. **Pradines, P., Brauner, M., Legrand, I., Sibony, M., and Garin, B.,** Letters. Heterotopic gastric mucosa in the gallbladder, *AJR*, 152, 432, 1989.
35. **Ralls, P. W., Mayekawa, D. S., Lee, K. P., Colletti, P. M., Johnson, M. B., and Halls, J. M.,** Gallbladder wall varices: diagnosis with color flow Doppler sonography, *J. Clin. Ultrasound*, 16, 595, 1988.

INDEX

I

J

L

M

N

O

P

W

Y

Z

G.T 19 No to F.4 18/01/06

Box Nos:- 5012, 5013, 5014, ~~5015,~~

27 64 60

Total Books:- 151

Total Boxes:- 3

AL 200